CONQUERING KIDNEY DISEASE

A Survivor's Guide to Thriving with CKD

James Fabin

Dadvice TV - Kidney Health Coach

Copyright © 2023 James Fabin

All rights reserved

No part of this book may be reproduced, or stored in a retrieval system, or transmitted in any form or by any means, electronic, mechanical, photocopying, recording, or otherwise, without express written permission of the publisher.

Paperback ISBN: 9798393242084
Hardcover ISBN: 9798394018497

Cover design by: James Fabin

Second Edition: May 2023

Limit of Liability/Disclaimer of Medical Advice

While the publisher and author have used their best efforts in writing and preparing this book, no representation or warranties exist with respect to the accuracy and completeness of this book, or that the contents apply to your current health or form of disease. The advice, research, diet, and plan may not be appropriate for all patients. A medical doctor should always assist you in making any treatment decisions, and patients should always be under the care and supervision of a physician. You should never make treatment decisions on your own without consulting a physician. Neither the author nor the publisher are liable for any medical decisions made based on the contents of this book. This includes special, incidental, consequential, or any other kinds of damages or liability.

Patients should always be under the care of a physician and defer to their physician for any and all treatment decisions. This book is not meant to replace a physician's advice, supervision, and counsel. No information in this book should be construed as medical advice. All medical decisions should be made by the patient and a qualified physician. This book is for informational purposes only.

This book is dedicated to all the kidney warriors I have had the privilege to meet and learn from during my journey. Your strength, resilience, and determination have inspired me, and your stories have left an indelible mark on my life. To those we have lost along the way, including John Vito, Russell Roberts, and Muriel Persaud, your memory continues to fuel my commitment to advocating for kidney health and supporting others in their battles against CKD. May this book serve as a beacon of hope and encouragement for kidney warriors everywhere, as we continue to fight together for a better tomorrow.

-James Fabin

CONTENTS

Title Page
Copyright
Dedication
Introduction
From Diagnosis to Triumph: My Battle with CKD — 1
My Strategy for Improving Kidney Function — 6
Kidneys 101 — 10
Introduction to Chronic Kidney Disease — 15
Diagnosing CKD — 20
CKD Stage 1 & Stage 2 — 25
CKD Stage 2: Mild Reduction in Kidney Function — 26
CKD Stage 3 — 29
CKD Stage 4 — 34
CKD Stage 5 - Navigating the Final Stage — 39
Causes and Risk Factors of CKD — 43
Heart Disease in CKD Patients — 47
Collaborating with Kidney Professionals — 50
Your First Kidney Doctor Visit — 57
Understanding Labs and Diagnostics — 60
Important Lab Test Values — 64
eGFR and Protein Leakage — 70

Reducing Protein in the Urine	74
Living with Chronic Kidney Disease	79
Lifestyle Changes to Slow CKD and Live Longer	83
Medications and Supplements for Kidney Health	86
The Latest Medications to Treat CKD	92
Emotional and Mental Health Support	99
Managing Co-Existing Conditions	104
The Importance of Blood Pressure Control	112
Creatinine and Your Kidneys	120
Is Kidney Failure in Your Future	122
Dialysis	125
Kidney Transplant	129
Tips for Finding an Organ Donor	135
Conservative Management of Kidney Failure	140
Diet and Nutrition for Kidney Health	145
Phosphorus	151
Potassium	157
Sodium	161
Protein and CKD	166
Fiber	170
Gut Health	174
The Kidney Diet: Foods to Watch	178
Starfruit and CKD - A Dangerous Combination	184
The Best Diet for CKD	187
Plant-Based is Not Vegetarian	192
Multivitamins for CKD Patients	195
7-Day Meal Plan Example (no restrictions)	200
7-Day Meal Plan Example (Potassium restriction)	203

Avoiding Common Diet Mistakes	206
Exercise and Physical Activity	209
Baking Soda and CKD	215
Anemia	220
Bubbles in Your Urine	224
Gout and Uric Acid	227
Kidney Stones	231
Itchy Skin and CKD	236
Sleepless Nights and Kidney Health	239
Understanding Kidney Pain	243
Life Expectancy of Those with CKD	247
Avoiding Kidney Myths and Scams	251
12 Bad Habits That Can Damage Your Kidneys	255
Unveiling My Secret to Kidney Success	258
Empowering Yourself Through Knowledge and Support	261
Glossary of Terms and Definitions	267
About The Author	277

INTRODUCTION

The journey through kidney disease is a challenging one, but it is not without hope or triumph. "Conquering Kidney Disease: A Survivor's Guide to Thriving with CKD" is a testament to the power of resilience, determination, and knowledge in the face of a life-altering diagnosis. This book is a compilation of invaluable insights and practical advice gleaned from my personal experience with chronic kidney disease (CKD), along with the wisdom of medical professionals, researchers, and fellow CKD warriors I have encountered along the way.

My own story began with a sudden and unexpected diagnosis of renal failure, which led me to confront the possibility of death and the harsh reality of dialysis. Unwilling to accept defeat, I embarked on a relentless quest for knowledge, seeking answers from experts around the world and exploring alternative approaches to CKD management. Through my research and unwavering determination, I discovered the transformative power of diet and lifestyle changes, which ultimately allowed me to regain control over my health and reclaim my life.

This book is divided into chapters that cover various aspects of living with CKD, from understanding the disease and its stages to managing dietary needs and coping with the emotional challenges that come with the diagnosis. Each chapter delves into essential topics, offering guidance and practical tips to help you navigate the complexities of CKD and improve your quality of life. In addition, we've included a comprehensive resource guide to support your continued learning and empower you to stay informed about the latest advancements in CKD care.

It is my sincerest hope that "Conquering Kidney Disease: A Survivor's Guide to Thriving with CKD" serves as a beacon of hope and inspiration for those facing the daunting reality of kidney disease. By sharing my story and the lessons I've learned, I aim to provide you with the tools and knowledge necessary to face CKD with courage, confidence, and optimism. Together, we can conquer kidney disease and emerge stronger, healthier, and more determined than ever before.

FROM DIAGNOSIS TO TRIUMPH: MY BATTLE WITH CKD

My CKD journey began with an unexpected twist that turned my life upside down. Little did I know that my kidneys were silently suffering, without any symptoms or warning signs. My story starts a year before my diagnosis, on a seemingly ordinary day. I was taking my kids and their grandpa out for ice cream when suddenly, a reckless driver ran an intersection and crashed into my SUV. The impact caused my vehicle to spin in the intersection before coming to a halt, facing the wrong direction. I was the last to be removed from my vehicle due to excruciating back pain, which marked the beginning of a long and arduous road to recovery.

Over the following 12 months, I underwent therapy to correct my spinal alignment, but the pain persisted. Lifting even common items or sitting for too long became excruciating. To cope with the back pain from my injuries, I relied on daily doses of Ibuprofen, always careful not to exceed the recommended dosage.

One fateful evening, while enjoying famous Cincinnati chili dogs with my family, I started to feel unwell. As the night wore on, my condition rapidly deteriorated. I felt increasingly worse, reminiscent of a past bout of food poisoning just days before my wedding. Over the next two weeks, my body betrayed me, unleashing a cascade of debilitating symptoms. My vision blurred, a persistent cough wracked my chest, and I suffered from throbbing headaches, teeth-rattling chills, itchy skin, and uncontrollable diarrhea. The simple act of eating became a torment, as constant vomiting wracked my weakened body. My energy dwindled, and I struggled to focus through the haze of an unrelenting headache. It felt as if death itself was knocking at my door, the toll of a merciless battle taking its toll on my very essence.

Unable to keep anything down, I would vomit up everything I tried to consume, even my life-sustaining blood pressure medication. The consequences were dire. My blood pressure skyrocketed dangerously, and I found myself teetering on the precipice of a life-threatening condition. Desperation and fear consumed me as I visited my family doctor, hoping for a shred of relief. To my dismay, the severity of my condition was immediately apparent to him. He wasted no time and insisted that I head straight to the emergency room. Although I initially hesitated, clinging to the idea of completing my daily errands, his stern warning left me no choice. I was confronted with the reality that every moment mattered, that my life hung in the balance.

Arriving at the emergency room, I mustered the last remnants of my waning energy. I was in a wheelchair, my strength sapped by the relentless assault on my body. Then, as if in a haze, I found myself on a stretcher, an IV needle piercing my arm. My arm, shoulder, and chest burned with an intensity that matched the inferno raging within. It was there, in the midst of the medical chaos, that the truth revealed itself with staggering clarity: my kidneys had failed, their once vibrant and vital function reduced to a mere flicker. With an eGFR of 8, the gravity of my situation unfolded before my disbelieving eyes when the Nephrologist told me I'd be dead within 45 days without dialysis.

The initial shock and fear were overwhelming. Questions flooded my mind, each more haunting than the last: What did dialysis mean for my future? How would it impact my daily life, my dreams, my aspirations? Was there a cure, a glimmer of hope in the darkness? And the thought that haunted me most: Would I be able to go home, to continue my work, to be there for my loved ones?

Determined to unravel the truth of my condition, I embarked on a relentless pursuit of knowledge. Hours upon hours were spent immersed in the depths of research, seeking answers, seeking solace. I discovered that kidney disease was not a death sentence, that other countries with fewer resources than my own were achieving better outcomes in kidney care. Their success hinged on a holistic approach, addressing diet, lifestyle changes, and medications to manage blood pressure and symptoms. It became painfully clear that my own country, the United States, lagged far behind in the quest for excellence in kidney care.

Despite the bleak prognosis delivered by my nephrologist, who insisted on dialysis, a glimmer of hope flickered deep within my soul. It was a hope nurtured by the research I had unearthed, by the stories of resilience and triumph that whispered in the dark corners of my mind. In that moment, I made a choice. **I chose to fight**, to fight kidney disease with every fiber of my being.

While in the ICU, my eGFR showed a slight improvement, but it remained perilously low. Dialysis loomed on the horizon, a formidable specter ready to claim me. However, I made a bold decision, fueled by a cocktail of hope and defiance. I refused to succumb to the fate prescribed by conventional wisdom. Instead, I embarked on a path less traveled, a path paved with dietary and lifestyle changes that promised a glimmer of salvation.

My journey to reclaim my health was not without its trials and tribulations. It required unwavering commitment, relentless discipline, and an unyielding spirit. With the guidance of my healthcare team, I discovered the perfect combination of blood pressure medications and implemented significant modifications to my diet. And as the days turned into weeks and the weeks into months, a miraculous transformation began to unfold. My eGFR climbed steadily, and with each passing day, my symptoms receded like shadows before the dawn. Energy surged through my veins, and I found myself walking five miles a day, a testament to the indomitable spirit within.

Throughout this challenging odyssey, I chronicled my experiences, my battles, my victories. My story became a beacon of hope, a source of solace for others navigating the treacherous waters of kidney disease. It was through the sharing of my journey that Dadvice TV was born, a platform that brought together individuals with kidney disease, healthcare professionals, and researchers. Together, we became a community, a force of resilience, and a source of knowledge. Dadvice TV became a sanctuary, a sanctuary of hope, compassion, and unwavering support.

Today, my website, DadviceTV.com, and my YouTube channel, Dadvice TV, serve as beacons of inspiration, reaching people across the globe. They provide a lifeline for those yearning for answers, for those desperate to regain control of their lives. My eGFR has stabilized in the low 30s, a testament to the power of determination and unwavering faith. I am now free from the shackles of debilitating symptoms, able to embrace life's myriad joys with unbridled enthusiasm. Together with my children, I explore new horizons, create cherished memories, and revel in the beauty of every precious moment.

Reflecting upon my journey, I have come to realize that the path to healing and resilience is rarely a solitary one. It is forged through the crucible of shared experiences, the unwavering support of loved ones, and the indomitable spirit that resides within each of us. My struggles have become a testament to the power of perseverance, hope, and the unbreakable bond of a compassionate community.

As a kidney health advocate, my purpose now is to illuminate the shadows of kidney disease, to raise awareness, and to empower others to seize control of their own destinies. I have undergone training to become a Kidney Health Coach through the American Kidney Fund, equipping me with additional tools to educate others about kidney disease. Through my story and the lessons learned on this extraordinary journey, I seek to inspire and ignite the flame of resilience within others. No one should face the trials of kidney disease alone. Together, we can weather the storm, triumph over adversity, and transform our lives.

My story is not one of mere survival; it is a testament to the remarkable resilience of the human spirit. I have emerged from the crucible of kidney disease stronger, more compassionate, and more determined than ever before. I am forever grateful for the opportunity to make a difference in the lives of those facing the same arduous journey. So, to all those who find themselves locked in a battle with kidney disease, I implore you to grasp the flickering torch of hope, to take charge of your destiny, and to march forward with unwavering resolve. You are not alone in this fight, for we stand together, a united front against the darkness. With every small victory, every hurdle overcome, we become living testaments to the triumph of the human spirit. We are warriors, capable of defying the odds and embracing life's grand tapestry with boundless joy. Together, let us walk this path of resilience, for it is paved with miracles waiting to unfold.

MY STRATEGY FOR IMPROVING KIDNEY FUNCTION

When faced with kidney failure and the discouraging prognosis that my condition would not improve, I decided to take control and implement changes that would positively impact my kidney health. With the support of my healthcare team, I managed to improve my kidney function from Stage 5 to Stage 3 without undergoing dialysis. In this chapter, I will share my personal strategy for enhancing kidney function.

Assembling a Supportive Healthcare Team

My journey began by seeking out a knowledgeable healthcare team with excellent communication skills. This team included my primary care physician and a dietitian well-versed in the latest research and treatments for kidney disease. Engaging in thorough and insightful conversations with my healthcare team enabled us to determine the most effective diet, medications, and lifestyle changes that would lead to improved kidney function.

Preventing Further Kidney Damage

Preserving kidney function requires halting any additional damage to the kidneys. This involves addressing the root cause of kidney disease and adopting a healthier lifestyle. For me, this entailed quitting smoking, limiting alcohol consumption, and managing my blood pressure and blood sugar levels. Even for those without diabetes, maintaining healthy blood sugar levels is crucial for individuals with chronic kidney disease (CKD).

Regularly Monitoring Labs

Blood work and urine analysis serve as essential guides for managing kidney disease. The objective is to maintain all results within the standard range. Dietitians utilize these labs to adjust your diet accordingly, helping to slow kidney function decline and manage or prevent symptoms. Regular monitoring is particularly important for individuals in Stage 4 or 5 kidney disease, as maintaining balance becomes increasingly difficult.

Taking Medications as Prescribed

Your healthcare team may prescribe medications to help manage kidney disease, symptoms, and other health issues. It is crucial to take these medications consistently and as prescribed. Using a free app or setting reminders can help ensure you never miss a dose.

Optimizing Nutrition Through Diet

Diet plays a crucial role in managing kidney disease, and optimizing your nutrition is essential for your overall well-being. To create a heart-healthy diet that's individualized for you, it's vital to consider your health, lifestyle, lab results, and personal nutritional needs. Instead of categorizing foods as simply good or bad, focus on finding a balance that meets your daily nutrient targets without overloading your body.

Guided by your lab results, pay attention to key nutrients such as phosphorus, potassium, sodium, protein, and sugar. Your healthcare team, including a renal dietitian, will assist you in making necessary diet modifications tailored to your individual needs. These personalized adjustments may include portion control, introducing more plant-based options, and emphasizing whole, nutrient-dense foods.

When creating your kidney-friendly diet, be mindful of your

choices and remember that it's essential not to make changes based solely on the experiences of other kidney patients. Each person's situation is unique, and what works for one individual may not be suitable for another. By focusing on your own nutritional requirements and working closely with your healthcare team, you can make informed decisions that support your kidney health and overall well-being.

Here is a form I use with my dietitian to set my daily nutritional targets:

	Daily Minimum		Daily Maximum	
Calories	_____		_____	
Calcium	_____	mg	_____	mg
Carbohydrates	_____	grams	_____	grams
Fiber	_____	grams	_____	grams
Iron	_____	mg	_____	mg
Protein	_____	grams	_____	grams
Phosphorus	_____	mg	_____	mg
Potassium	_____	mg	_____	mg
Sodium	_____	mg	_____	mg
Water	_____	ounces	_____	ounces
Avoid:	_____
Limit:	_____

Using Supplements Correctly

Your healthcare team may recommend supplements to address dietary deficiencies. However, it is vital only to take supplements prescribed by your healthcare team, as self-prescribing can lead to kidney damage, medication interference, and other health issues.

Staying Active

Most doctors recommend at least 30 minutes of low-impact activity five days a week for kidney patients. This can include walking, dancing, or playing a sport. Staying active helps maintain a healthy weight, manage blood pressure and blood sugar, and support mental health.

Managing Weight

Many transplant centers require a body mass index (BMI) of 30 or better. By working towards a healthier weight, you can improve your overall health and be prepared should you need a transplant in the future. Set realistic goals for reaching a BMI of 35, then 30, and finally, 25.

Managing Stress

Finding healthy ways to relax and avoiding negative influences are essential for managing stress. Chronic stress can strain your body, hinder your diet, and prevent kidney function improvement. By following your healthcare team's recommendations and adhering to your prescribed diet, you can help alleviate stress on your kidneys.

Educating Yourself on Kidney Disease

Knowledge is power, and understanding kidney disease is crucial for managing your condition. Educating yourself enables you to have better conversations with your healthcare team, reduce stress and anxiety, and allows you to be proactive in your care and treatment strategy. Let's now get started understanding kidney disease!

KIDNEYS 101

Kidneys: The Unsung Heroes of Overall Health

Kidneys are vital organs that play a pivotal role in maintaining overall health. While they often take a backseat in discussions about the human body, their importance is undeniable. In this chapter, we will explore the various functions of the kidneys and how they contribute to overall health. By understanding the role of the kidneys, you can better appreciate their significance and the need to maintain their health.

Anatomy and Location: The Kidneys' Strategic Position

The human body has two kidneys, which are bean-shaped organs, each roughly the size of a fist. They are strategically located on either side of the spine, just below the rib cage, in the lower back region. Each kidney is composed of approximately 1 million tiny filtering units called nephrons. Nephrons are the functional units of the kidneys responsible for filtering waste products, excess water, and toxins from the blood, playing a central role in maintaining a healthy internal environment.

Blood Supply and Nephrons: A Dynamic Partnership

The kidneys filter all of the blood in your body several times a day, making them one of the most highly perfused organs in the body. Blood enters each kidney through the renal artery, which branches into smaller arteries, eventually reaching the nephrons. As blood flows through the nephrons, waste products, excess water, and toxins are filtered out, while essential nutrients and electrolytes are reabsorbed into the bloodstream. The filtered waste products, water, and toxins form urine, which then flows through the renal tubules and collecting ducts into the renal pelvis. From the renal pelvis, urine is transported to the bladder via the ureters, where it is stored until it is eliminated from the body through the urethra.

The Multifaceted Functions of the Kidneys

The kidneys perform a variety of essential functions that contribute to overall health. These functions include:

Filtering Waste Products and Toxins: The primary function of the kidneys is to filter waste products and toxins from the blood, which are then excreted through the urine. This process helps maintain the balance of chemicals and fluids in the body, ensuring a healthy internal environment.

Regulating Fluid Balance: Kidneys help maintain the balance of fluids in the body by adjusting the amount of water that is reabsorbed into the bloodstream or excreted as urine. This balance is crucial for proper hydration, blood pressure control, and overall health.

Electrolyte Balance: The kidneys play a critical role in maintaining the balance of electrolytes in the body, including sodium, potassium, calcium, and phosphate. Electrolytes are essential for various body functions, including muscle contractions, nerve transmissions, and maintaining the body's acid-base balance.

Acid-Base Balance: The kidneys help maintain the body's acid-base balance by excreting excess acids or bases in the urine. This balance is critical for maintaining the proper pH of blood and other body fluids, which is essential for optimal functioning of cells, tissues, and organs.

Hormone Production: The kidneys produce several hormones that are essential for various body functions. Some of these hormones include:

- Erythropoietin (EPO): This hormone stimulates the production of red blood cells in the bone marrow, which helps maintain an adequate supply of oxygen-carrying cells in the bloodstream.
- Renin: This enzyme is involved in regulating blood pressure by controlling the constriction and dilation of blood vessels.
- Calcitriol (active vitamin D): This hormone helps regulate calcium and phosphate balance, which is essential for bone health and overall mineral balance in the body.

Blood Pressure Regulation: The kidneys play a crucial role in regulating blood pressure by managing the volume and composition of bodily fluids, as well as producing hormones that influence blood vessel constriction and dilation. In later chapters, we will explore how high blood pressure is a primary cause of kidney damage, which in turn impairs the kidney's ability to regulate blood pressure effectively. This creates a snowball effect, causing the kidneys to deteriorate progressively, ultimately leading to kidney failure.

Glucose Homeostasis: The kidneys help maintain blood glucose levels by reabsorbing filtered glucose and producing glucose through a process called gluconeogenesis. This helps ensure that the body has a constant supply of energy, particularly during periods of fasting or intense physical activity.

Metabolism of Medications: The kidneys play a significant role in the metabolism and elimination of medications from the body. They help filter out drugs and their metabolites, ensuring that the body is not exposed to potentially harmful substances for extended periods.

Urea Production: The kidneys produce urea, a waste product formed from the breakdown of proteins in the liver. Urea is then transported to the kidneys, where it is filtered and excreted in the urine.

The Critical Importance of Kidney Health

Preserving the health of our kidneys is crucial for overall well-being. Kidney disease or malfunction can give rise to an array of complications, such as:

Fluid Overload: When kidneys cannot effectively regulate fluid balance, excess fluid may accumulate within the body. This can result in swelling (edema), elevated blood pressure, and potentially fatal conditions like congestive heart failure.

Electrolyte Imbalances: Compromised kidney function can lead to imbalances in critical electrolytes, including potassium and sodium. This may cause muscle weakness, irregular heartbeats, and additional complications.

Anemia: Damaged kidneys can produce less erythropoietin, resulting in anemia. This condition is marked by a decline in red blood cell count and a diminished capacity to transport oxygen throughout the body.

Bone and Mineral Disorders: Impaired kidney function can upset the balance of calcium and phosphate, causing weakened bones, an increased likelihood of fractures, and other complications related to bone and mineral metabolism.

Cardiovascular Disease: The risk of cardiovascular disease escalates in the presence of kidney disease, owing to factors such as hypertension, fluid overload, and the accumulation of detrimental substances in the bloodstream.

Kidney Failure: Severe kidney disease can culminate in kidney failure, a life-threatening condition where the kidneys can no longer carry out their essential functions. Treatment options for kidney failure include dialysis or a kidney transplant.

The Kidney Lingo

As a kidney patient, you'll encounter a whole new world of kidney-related terminology. This book includes a comprehensive section on common kidney terms to help you navigate the language of kidney health with ease. To start, it's essential to understand that the words "Nephrology," "Renal," and "Kidney" are entirely interchangeable. These three terms all refer to the same thing, so you'll often see them used in various contexts throughout your kidney health journey.

INTRODUCTION TO CHRONIC KIDNEY DISEASE

Understanding Chronic Kidney Disease and Acute Kidney Injury

Chronic Kidney Disease (CKD) is a long-term health condition that impacts a significant number of individuals across the globe. It involves the slow and steady decline of kidney function, which can result in a range of health issues and eventually necessitate dialysis or a kidney transplant. In this chapter, we'll cover the basics of CKD, how common it is, the risks connected to it, and why early detection, treatment, and teamwork are essential.

Acute Kidney Injury (AKI) is a sudden and temporary decline in kidney function that can occur over a short period of time, typically within a few hours or days. It is often caused by factors such as dehydration, infections, or exposure to certain medications or toxins. It is important to note that it is possible to have both AKI and CKD simultaneously. In such cases, once the AKI is addressed and resolved, the individual may see an improvement in their kidney function. However, this improvement does not mean that their CKD has been cured. They would still have CKD and need to continue monitoring and managing their kidney health, as the underlying chronic condition remains.

Prevalence and Impact of CKD

According to the Centers for Disease Control and Prevention (CDC), approximately 15% of adults in the United States, or about 37 million people, are estimated to have CKD[1]. However, 9 out of 10 people with CKD are unaware of their condition, highlighting the importance of early detection and intervention[1]. Globally, the prevalence of CKD is also significant. A study published in The Lancet estimates that 9.1% of the world's population, or roughly 700 million people, are affected by CKD[2]. It is the 12th leading cause of death worldwide and contributes to an estimated 1.2 million deaths annually[2].

CKD is often referred to as a "silent" disease because it frequently progresses without noticeable symptoms until the later stages (commonly stages 4 & 5). This lack of overt symptoms makes early diagnosis challenging, leading to delayed treatment and a higher risk of severe complications. Consequently, CKD is recognized as a major public health issue and a leading cause of morbidity and mortality worldwide.

The economic burden of CKD is substantial, with healthcare systems around the world spending billions annually on CKD-related care. The costs associated with CKD encompass direct medical expenses, such as hospitalizations, dialysis, and medications, as well as indirect costs tied to lost productivity and disability. As the prevalence of CKD continues to climb, so does its economic impact, emphasizing the need for increased awareness, early detection, and effective management strategies.

The Progression of CKD

CKD is a progressive disease, meaning it worsens over time as kidney function deteriorates. The progression of CKD is categorized into five stages based on the level of kidney function, as measured by the estimated glomerular filtration rate (eGFR). The eGFR is a calculation that estimates the volume of blood filtered by the kidneys per minute and is derived from blood tests measuring waste product levels, such as creatinine. Think of eGFR as your Kidney Function number – the higher it is, the better your kidneys are functioning.

The five stages of CKD are as follows:

Stage 1: Normal kidney function (eGFR ≥ 90) with evidence of kidney damage

Stage 2: Mildly reduced kidney function (eGFR 60-89) with evidence of kidney damage

Stage 3: Moderately reduced kidney function, divided into two sub-stages: Stage 3a (eGFR 45-59) and Stage 3b (eGFR 30-44)

Stage 4: Severely reduced kidney function (eGFR 15-29)

Stage 5: Kidney failure, also known as end-stage renal disease (ESRD) (eGFR <15)

In CKD's early stages, kidney function may be only mildly reduced, and individuals may not experience any noticeable symptoms. However, as the disease progresses and kidney function declines, various complications and health issues can emerge. These complications include fluid retention, electrolyte imbalances, anemia, bone disorders, cardiovascular disease, and nerve damage. It's essential to manage CKD early to slow its progression and reduce the risk of these complications.

The Importance of Early Detection and Management

Considering the potentially severe complications associated with CKD and the disease's silent nature, early detection and proactive management are crucial. Identifying CKD in its early stages allows for timely intervention and implementation of strategies to slow the disease's progression, reduce the risk of complications, and enhance overall health.

Effective management of CKD involves addressing the

underlying causes of the disease, such as controlling blood sugar levels in individuals with diabetes and managing blood pressure in those with hypertension. Additionally, adopting a healthy lifestyle, including maintaining a balanced diet, engaging in regular physical activity, and avoiding tobacco use, can help slow CKD's progression and improve overall health.

In more advanced stages of CKD, medical interventions such as medications, dialysis, or kidney transplantation may be necessary to manage the disease and its complications. However, even in these advanced stages, maintaining a healthy lifestyle and working closely with a healthcare team can improve the quality of life and potentially extend life expectancy.

Monitoring and Screening for CKD

Regular monitoring and screening for CKD are essential, particularly for individuals at higher risk of developing the disease, such as those with a family history of kidney disease, diabetes, or hypertension. Routine blood and urine tests can help detect early signs of kidney damage and reduced kidney function, enabling healthcare providers to implement appropriate interventions and management strategies.

Collaborative Care for CKD Patients

Managing CKD effectively requires a collaborative approach involving healthcare professionals from various disciplines. A team consisting of primary care physicians (your regular doctor), nephrologists (kidney doctor), dietitians, and other specialists can work together to create a personalized care plan for each CKD patient. This care plan may encompass medical treatments, lifestyle modifications, and ongoing monitoring of kidney function and overall health. Patients are encouraged to actively participate in their care and communicate openly with their healthcare team to ensure the best possible outcomes.

References:

[1]Centers for Disease Control and Prevention (CDC). (2021). Chronic Kidney Disease in the United States, 2021. [online] Available at: https://www.cdc.gov/kidneydisease/pdf/CKD-Factsheet_2021-508.pdf

[2]GBD Chronic Kidney Disease Collaboration. (2020). Global, regional, and national burden of chronic kidney disease, 1990–2017: a systematic analysis for the Global Burden of Disease Study 2017. The Lancet, 395(102 25), pp.709-733. [online] Available at: https://www.thelancet.com/journals/lancet/article/PIIS0140-6736(20)30045-3/fulltext

DIAGNOSING CKD

Early detection and accurate diagnosis of chronic kidney disease (CKD) are essential for managing the condition effectively and preventing or delaying the onset of severe complications. In this chapter, we will discuss the various tests and diagnostic tools used to identify CKD and the criteria required to confirm a CKD diagnosis.

Screening for CKD

Screening for Chronic Kidney Disease (CKD) is a crucial step in identifying the condition early and initiating appropriate interventions. It involves the use of specific tests to assess kidney function and detect any abnormalities. Certain individuals are at a higher risk of developing CKD and should undergo regular screening. This includes individuals with:

- **Diabetes**: Diabetes is a leading cause of kidney disease. People with diabetes should be screened annually for CKD, starting from the time of diagnosis.
- **Hypertension**: High blood pressure is both a risk factor and a consequence of CKD. Individuals with hypertension should be screened regularly to monitor kidney function. *[handwritten note: I wasn't screened for this →]*
- **Family history**: If you have a close relative with CKD, you may have an increased risk and should consider screening.
- **Age**: As we age, the risk of developing kidney disease increases. Regular screening is recommended for individuals over the age of 60.

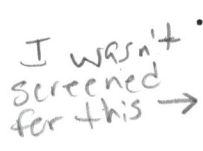

- **Other conditions**: Certain medical conditions, such as cardiovascular disease, obesity, autoimmune diseases, and urinary tract abnormalities, may increase the risk of CKD and warrant screening.

Diagnostic Tests for CKD

Several tests can help healthcare providers identify and assess kidney function, damage, and potential underlying causes of CKD. These tests include:

Blood tests:

- Serum creatinine: Serum creatinine is a waste product produced by muscle metabolism and is cleared by the kidneys. Elevated levels of serum creatinine indicate reduced kidney function. This test helps estimate the glomerular filtration rate (GFR), a measure of how well the kidneys are functioning. Higher creatinine levels and lower GFR values indicate poorer kidney function.

- Blood urea nitrogen (BUN): BUN is a measure of the amount of urea nitrogen in the blood. Elevated BUN levels can indicate impaired kidney function, but it can also be influenced by other factors such as dehydration or a high-protein diet.

- Electrolyte levels: Blood tests can assess electrolyte levels, such as sodium, potassium, and bicarbonate, which can become imbalanced in CKD.

Urine tests:

- Urinalysis: Urinalysis involves analyzing a urine sample for the presence of protein, blood, or other substances. Proteinuria (excessive protein in the urine) is a hallmark sign of kidney damage or dysfunction.

- Albumin-to-creatinine ratio (ACR): This test quantifies the amount of albumin (a type of protein) in the urine relative to the creatinine level. Elevated ACR values indicate proteinuria and can help determine the extent of kidney damage.

Imaging tests:

- Ultrasound: Ultrasound imaging uses sound waves to produce images of the kidneys. It can help detect abnormalities in the size, shape, or structure of the kidneys, such as cysts or tumors.
- CT scan or MRI: These imaging techniques may be used in specific cases to provide more detailed information about the kidneys and surrounding structures.

Kidney biopsy:

In some cases, a kidney biopsy may be performed to obtain a small sample of kidney tissue for analysis. This procedure is typically reserved for situations where the cause or extent of kidney damage needs further evaluation.

Other tests:

Depending on the specific circumstances and suspected causes of CKD, additional tests may be recommended. These tests can include genetic testing, autoimmune markers, or specialized blood tests to assess specific kidney-related conditions.

Criteria for CKD Diagnosis

To confirm a CKD diagnosis, healthcare providers typically

use the following criteria:

- Persistent kidney damage: Kidney damage can be assessed through various methods, such as the presence of proteinuria (excessive protein in the urine) or abnormal imaging findings. Persistent kidney damage refers to the sustained presence of these abnormalities over a period of at least three months.
- Decreased kidney function: Decreased kidney function is determined by estimating the glomerular filtration rate (GFR), which reflects how well the kidneys are filtering waste from the blood. A GFR below 60 for three months or longer indicates decreased kidney function and is a criterion for CKD diagnosis.

It is important to note that a single test result **does not** necessarily indicate the presence of CKD. Kidney function can fluctuate due to various factors, such as dehydration or certain medications, which can temporarily affect test results. Therefore, a diagnosis of CKD requires the persistence of kidney damage and decreased kidney function over time.

Dehydration can lead to a temporary decrease in kidney function, resulting in elevated creatinine levels and reduced GFR. In such cases, rehydration and subsequent repeat testing may show improved kidney function. It is crucial to ensure proper hydration before interpreting test results.

Certain medications, such as nonsteroidal anti-inflammatory drugs (NSAIDs) or certain antibiotics, can also affect kidney function and test results. These medications may cause acute kidney injury, which is a reversible condition. However, in some cases, continued use or misuse of medications can lead to chronic kidney damage. It is important to discuss any medications or supplements you are taking with your healthcare provider to ensure they are safe for your kidneys and do not interfere with diagnostic tests.

The diagnosis of CKD requires a comprehensive evaluation that considers clinical presentation, medical history, laboratory tests, and imaging findings. It is crucial to work closely with your healthcare team, including nephrologists and primary care physicians, who can interpret the test results in the context of your overall health and guide you through the diagnostic process.

CKD STAGE 1 & STAGE 2

In the early stages of chronic kidney disease (CKD), individuals may not experience any noticeable symptoms, making it challenging to identify the condition without proper testing. However, understanding the characteristics and implications of Stage 1 and Stage 2 CKD is crucial for managing the disease and adopting a healthy lifestyle to prevent or delay its progression. In this chapter, we will discuss Stage 1 and Stage 2 CKD, emphasizing the importance of maintaining kidney health and addressing underlying health conditions.

CKD Stage 1: The Beginning

Stage 1 CKD is characterized by normal or only slightly reduced kidney function (eGFR ≥ 90) with evidence of kidney damage. Although kidney function remains relatively normal during this stage, early signs of kidney damage, such as protein in the urine or structural abnormalities, may be present.

It is essential to understand that, despite the lack of symptoms, Stage 1 CKD should be taken seriously. At this stage, individuals should focus on identifying and addressing any underlying conditions or lifestyle factors contributing to kidney damage. This could include controlling blood pressure and blood sugar, maintaining a healthy weight, and avoiding tobacco use. While there are no diet restrictions with Stage 1, it's a good time to make sure you are eating heart-healthy.

CKD STAGE 2: MILD REDUCTION IN KIDNEY FUNCTION

Stage 2 CKD is marked by a mildly reduced kidney function (eGFR 60-89) with evidence of kidney damage (such as protein in your urine). Like Stage 1, individuals with Stage 2 CKD most likely won't experience any noticeable symptoms, but kidney damage is still present.

At this stage, the importance of adopting a healthy lifestyle and addressing underlying health conditions becomes even more critical. Maintaining a heart-healthy balanced diet, engaging in regular physical activity, and working closely with healthcare providers to manage conditions such as hypertension and diabetes can help slow the progression of CKD.

Living with Stage 1 and Stage 2 CKD

Although the early stages of CKD may not cause any noticeable symptoms, individuals should not ignore their diagnosis. Instead, they should use this as motivation to make necessary lifestyle changes and prioritize their kidney health. By adopting a healthy lifestyle and addressing underlying health conditions, individuals with Stage 1 and Stage 2 CKD can potentially maintain their kidney function and prevent further progression for the rest of their natural lives.

Key Steps to Preserve Kidney Health in Early CKD

Regular monitoring: Work closely with healthcare providers to monitor kidney function and underlying health conditions regularly. This will enable timely detection of any changes in kidney function and allow for appropriate adjustments in treatment or lifestyle.

Blood pressure control: High blood pressure is a leading cause of CKD. Keeping blood pressure within a healthy range can help protect the kidneys from further damage.

Blood sugar management: For individuals with diabetes, maintaining healthy blood sugar levels is essential in preventing or slowing the progression of CKD.

Healthy diet: Adopting a balanced, kidney-friendly diet can help protect kidney function. This may involve reducing sodium intake, moderating protein consumption, and focusing on nutrient-dense foods.

Physical activity: Regular physical activity can help maintain a healthy weight, lower blood pressure, and improve overall health, all of which benefit kidney function.

Avoiding nephrotoxic substances: Some medications and substances can be harmful to the kidneys. Speak with a healthcare provider before taking any new medications or supplements, and avoid excessive use of over-the-counter pain relievers such as NSAIDs (aspirin, ibuprofen, naproxen, etc.).

Avoid smoking: Tobacco use is harmful to the kidneys and can exacerbate the progression of CKD. Quitting smoking can significantly benefit kidney health and overall well-being.

Stage 1 and Stage 2 CKD may not cause noticeable symptoms, but understanding and addressing these early stages is crucial in preserving kidney function and maintaining overall health. By using the diagnosis as a motivator to adopt a healthier lifestyle and prioritize kidney health, individuals can potentially slow down or even halt the progression of CKD.

Awareness and education about the early stages of CKD

are crucial in promoting kidney health and preventing further damage. It is essential to work closely with healthcare providers to monitor kidney function, manage underlying health conditions, and develop a personalized care plan tailored to individual needs.

CKD STAGE 3

Stage 3 Chronic Kidney Disease (CKD) is a crucial point in the progression of kidney disease, as it marks the transition from mild to moderate kidney damage. At this stage, the estimated glomerular filtration rate (eGFR) falls between 30 and 59, indicating a moderate reduction in kidney function. Although most people do not experience noticeable symptoms at this stage, it is essential to be vigilant and proactive in managing CKD to slow its progression and minimize the risk of complications.

Potential Symptoms in Stage 3 CKD

While many people with Stage 3 CKD do not experience noticeable symptoms, some individuals may begin to notice subtle changes in their health. Possible symptoms that may arise during Stage 3 CKD, especially as you near Stage 4, include:

- Fatigue and weakness
- Swelling in the hands, feet, or face (edema)
- Changes in urine color, frequency, or appearance (such as foamy or bubbly urine)
- Back or flank pain (very rare this is actually caused by kidney disease at this stage)
- Changes in appetite or taste
- Difficulty concentrating or memory problems
- Sleep disturbances, such as insomnia or sleep apnea
- Itchy or dry skin

It is important to remember that these symptoms can also be associated with other medical conditions or lifestyle factors. If you experience any of these symptoms, consult your healthcare provider to determine their cause and receive appropriate care.

The Role of Nephrologists and Renal Dietitians in Stage 3 CKD Management

Stage 3 CKD is typically the point at which individuals are referred to a nephrologist, a kidney specialist, for more specialized care. Nephrologists have extensive expertise in diagnosing and managing kidney diseases and can help guide individuals through the process of optimizing their kidney health.

In addition to working with a nephrologist, individuals with Stage 3 CKD can greatly benefit from consulting with a renal dietitian. Renal dietitians specialize in creating personalized nutrition plans for individuals with kidney disease, focusing on a heart-healthy diet that reduces the burden on the kidneys and slows the progression of kidney disease. By working with a renal dietitian, individuals can gain a deeper understanding of the role nutrition plays in kidney health and receive guidance on how to make informed dietary choices that support their overall well-being.

Managing Blood Pressure and Blood Sugar

Blood pressure and blood sugar control are of paramount importance in managing Stage 3 CKD. Uncontrolled hypertension (high blood pressure) and hyperglycemia (high blood sugar) can place additional stress on the kidneys, accelerating the progression of kidney disease. Therefore, it is crucial for individuals with CKD to work closely with their healthcare providers to develop a comprehensive plan for managing these conditions, including medication management, dietary modifications, and lifestyle changes.

Key Steps to Preserve Kidney Health with CKD Stage 3

1. **Regular monitoring**: Schedule regular appointments with your healthcare provider and nephrologist to monitor your kidney function, blood pressure, and blood sugar levels. This will help ensure that any changes in your condition are promptly addressed and managed.

2. **Follow a kidney-friendly diet**: Consult with a renal dietitian to develop a personalized meal plan that supports kidney health. This may include limiting sodium and phosphorus intake, consuming an appropriate amount of protein, and focusing on heart-healthy foods like fruits, vegetables, and whole grains. Don't worry – your diet isn't going to be very restrictive, but it is going to be healthy. As you approach the next stage, restrictions may start to be recommended by your healthcare team or dietitian.

3. **Manage blood pressure**: Maintain healthy blood pressure levels through a combination of medication, diet, and lifestyle modifications. This may involve reducing sodium intake, increasing physical activity, maintaining a healthy weight, and managing stress.

4. **Control blood sugar**: If you have diabetes, work closely with your healthcare team to develop a comprehensive plan for managing your blood sugar levels. This may include medication, insulin therapy, dietary adjustments, and regular glucose monitoring.

5. **Stay physically active**: Engage in regular physical activity, such as walking, swimming, or cycling,

to help maintain a healthy weight, improve cardiovascular health, and support overall kidney function.

6. **Avoid smoking and limit alcohol consumption**: Smoking and excessive alcohol consumption can increase the risk of kidney damage and cardiovascular disease. Quitting smoking and limiting alcohol intake are essential steps in preserving kidney health.

7. **Use medications cautiously**: Some medications, particularly nonsteroidal anti-inflammatory drugs (NSAIDs), can harm your kidneys if taken in high doses or over an extended period. Discuss your medications with your healthcare provider to ensure they are safe for your kidneys and follow their recommendations for use.

8. **Stay hydrated**: Drinking an adequate amount of water helps your kidneys flush out waste products and maintain proper fluid balance. Talk to your healthcare provider about the appropriate amount of fluids you should consume daily.

9. **Manage underlying health conditions**: If you have other health conditions that can impact kidney health, such as high cholesterol, heart disease, or autoimmune diseases, work with your healthcare provider to manage these conditions effectively.

10. **Educate yourself and stay informed**: Learn as much as you can about CKD and kidney health, as this will empower you to make informed decisions about your care and actively participate in your treatment plan.

By following these key steps and working closely with your healthcare team, you can take control of your CKD Stage 3 and work towards preserving your kidney function and overall health.

CKD STAGE 4

Chronic Kidney Disease (CKD) Stage 4 is a crucial phase in the progression of kidney disease, as it marks a significant decline in kidney function. This stage is characterized by an estimated glomerular filtration rate (eGFR) of 15-29, which indicates that the kidneys are operating at less than 30% of their normal capacity. As kidney function continues to decline, it becomes increasingly vital for individuals to prioritize their health and make the necessary lifestyle changes to manage their condition effectively. In this chapter, we will discuss the symptoms, challenges, and key strategies for living with CKD Stage 4.

Symptoms of CKD Stage 4

While some people may not experience any noticeable symptoms, others may begin to experience a range of signs and symptoms associated with reduced kidney function. These can include:

- Fatigue and weakness
- Swelling in the hands, feet, or face (edema)
- Shortness of breath
- Changes in urine output, including foamy or dark-colored urine
- Nausea and vomiting
- Loss of appetite
- Difficulty concentrating or confusion
- Itching or dry skin

- Sleep disturbances, such as insomnia or restless leg syndrome
- Bone or joint pain

Life with CKD Stage 4

Living with CKD Stage 4 can present several challenges, as individuals must adapt to their changing health status and learn to manage their condition effectively. This may involve closely monitoring their kidney function, making significant dietary and lifestyle adjustments, and working with a team of healthcare professionals to ensure optimal care and support.

Managing Blood Pressure

Controlling blood pressure is crucial in CKD Stage 4, as high blood pressure can further damage the kidneys and contribute to the progression of kidney disease. Strategies for managing blood pressure may include:

- Taking prescribed blood pressure medications as directed by your healthcare provider
- Limiting sodium intake and following a low-sodium diet
- Maintaining a healthy weight through a balanced diet and regular physical activity
- Reducing stress and incorporating stress management techniques, such as meditation or deep breathing exercises
- Avoiding tobacco use and limiting alcohol consumption

Eating a Kidney-Friendly Diet

A kidney-friendly diet is essential in managing CKD Stage 4, as it can help alleviate some symptoms, slow the progression of kidney disease, and promote overall health. Key aspects of a kidney-friendly diet may include:

- Limiting sodium, potassium, and phosphorus intake per your dietitian's recommendations
- Consuming an appropriate amount of high-quality protein
- Focusing on heart-healthy foods, such as fruits, vegetables, whole grains, and lean proteins
- Avoiding processed and high-sodium foods
- Consulting with a renal dietitian to develop a personalized meal plan

Living a Healthy Lifestyle

Adopting a healthy lifestyle is paramount in CKD Stage 4, as it can help improve overall health, support kidney function, and enhance the quality of life. Key components of a healthy lifestyle may include:

- Engaging in regular physical activity, such as walking, swimming, or cycling, to promote cardiovascular health and maintain a healthy weight
- Practicing good sleep hygiene and addressing any sleep disturbances
- Staying well-hydrated by drinking an appropriate amount of fluids as recommended by your healthcare provider
- Participating in stress reduction activities, such as yoga, meditation, or mindfulness exercises
- Seeking support from friends, family, or support groups to help navigate the challenges of living with CKD Stage 4

The Importance of Taking Action

While it is essential to maintain a positive outlook, it is also crucial to recognize the seriousness of CKD Stage 4 and take the necessary steps to manage the condition effectively. If you have not already made significant lifestyle changes to support your kidney health, **now is the time** to take action.

Working with a Team of Healthcare Professionals

A comprehensive healthcare team is vital for individuals with CKD Stage 4, as they can provide the necessary guidance, support, and medical interventions to manage the condition effectively. Your healthcare team may include:

- Nephrologist: A kidney specialist who will monitor your kidney function, prescribe medications, and manage any complications related to CKD.
- Renal Dietitian: A nutrition expert who can help you develop a personalized kidney-friendly meal plan and provide dietary advice tailored to your specific needs.
- Primary Care Physician: A healthcare provider who can coordinate your overall care and address any additional health concerns that may arise.
- Nurse: A healthcare professional who can assist with medication management, provide education about CKD, and offer support and resources.
- Mental Health Professional: A therapist, psychologist, or counselor who can help you cope with the emotional challenges of living with CKD Stage 4 and provide strategies for managing stress and anxiety.

Living with CKD Stage 4 presents several challenges, but with the right approach, it is possible to manage the condition effectively, slow its progression, and maintain a good quality of life. Prioritizing blood pressure management, adopting a kidney-friendly diet, and embracing a healthy lifestyle are key strategies for preserving kidney health and overall well-being. Working closely with a team of healthcare professionals and making the necessary lifestyle changes can empower you to take control of your CKD journey and navigate life with confidence and resilience.

CKD STAGE 5 - NAVIGATING THE FINAL STAGE

Chronic Kidney Disease (CKD) Stage 5, also known as end-stage renal disease (ESRD), is the final stage of kidney disease where kidney function is severely reduced or lost entirely. At this stage, the kidneys are unable to perform their essential functions, and individuals may require renal replacement therapy, such as dialysis or a kidney transplant. However, it is important to note that not all patients with CKD Stage 5 will require dialysis immediately. The initiation of dialysis depends on a variety of factors, including estimated glomerular filtration rate (eGFR), symptoms, and other risk factors that cannot be managed effectively. In this chapter, we will discuss CKD Stage 5 in detail, including the symptoms, treatment options, and considerations for initiating dialysis.

Symptoms of CKD Stage 5

As kidney function declines further in Stage 5, individuals may experience a range of symptoms and complications, including:

- Fatigue and weakness
- Nausea and vomiting
- Loss of appetite and weight loss
- Swelling in the hands, feet, and face (edema)

- Shortness of breath
- Difficulty concentrating and confusion
- Metallic taste in the mouth or bad breath
- Itching and dry skin
- Muscle cramps and restless legs
- Sleep disturbances, such as insomnia or sleep apnea
- Changes in urine output and color
- Anemia

Initiating Dialysis in CKD Stage 5

Contrary to popular belief, dialysis **does not** automatically begin when a patient reaches CKD Stage 5. The decision to start dialysis is typically based on a combination of factors, such as the patient's eGFR, symptoms, and overall health. Generally, the current standard for initiating dialysis is when the eGFR falls between 5 and 7 unless there are other risk factors or symptoms that cannot be effectively managed. Some factors that may prompt earlier initiation of dialysis include:

- Severe fluid overload that does not respond to diuretics
- Life-threatening electrolyte imbalances, such as high potassium levels
- Severe acidosis
- Significant decline in nutritional status
- Persistent and severe symptoms affecting the patient's quality of life

Treatment Options for CKD Stage 5

When managing CKD Stage 5, the primary goal is to alleviate symptoms, maintain the patient's quality of life, and, if necessary, initiate renal replacement therapy. Treatment options for CKD Stage 5 include:

- Dialysis: There are two main types of dialysis – hemodialysis and peritoneal dialysis. Hemodialysis uses a machine to filter waste products and excess fluids from the blood, while peritoneal dialysis uses the lining of the abdomen (peritoneum) as a natural filter. The choice of dialysis modality depends on factors such as the patient's overall health, lifestyle, and personal preferences.

- Kidney Transplant: A kidney transplant involves surgically replacing the damaged kidneys with a healthy kidney from a living or deceased donor. While a kidney transplant can significantly improve the patient's quality of life and offer a longer life expectancy compared to dialysis, it is not a suitable option for everyone. Factors such as age, overall health, and the availability of a suitable donor can affect eligibility for a transplant.

- Conservative Management: For some patients, particularly older individuals or those with multiple health issues, conservative management may be an appropriate option. This approach focuses on managing symptoms and complications of CKD Stage 5 without dialysis or transplantation. It may include medical interventions, dietary modifications, and supportive care to optimize the patient's quality of life.

Maintaining a Healthy Lifestyle in CKD Stage 5

Even in CKD Stage 5, it is crucial to maintain a healthy lifestyle and manage any underlying health conditions, such as high blood pressure or diabetes. Key aspects of a healthy lifestyle in CKD Stage 5 include:

1. Dietary Management: A renal dietitian can help

tailor a personalized meal plan that meets the patient's nutritional needs while managing the complications of CKD. The diet may involve controlling protein, sodium, potassium, and phosphorus intake, depending on the patient's individual requirements.

2. Blood Pressure Control: Managing blood pressure is essential in CKD Stage 5 to slow the progression of kidney disease and reduce the risk of cardiovascular complications. This may involve taking prescribed medications, maintaining a low-sodium diet, and engaging in regular physical activity.

3. Blood Sugar Control: For patients with diabetes, your healthcare team may be more relaxed in how tightly they control your blood sugar to minimize the risk of additional complications.

4. Physical Activity: Engaging in regular physical activity, as recommended by a healthcare provider, can help improve overall health, manage symptoms, and maintain a healthy body weight.

5. Medication Management: Taking prescribed medications as directed and attending regular follow-up appointments with healthcare providers can help manage the symptoms and complications of CKD Stage 5.

CAUSES AND RISK FACTORS OF CKD

Understanding the causes and risk factors of chronic kidney disease (CKD) is essential for preventing its onset and managing its progression effectively. In this chapter, we will discuss the various causes and risk factors associated with CKD to help individuals take preventive measures and maintain their kidney health.

Causes of CKD

There are several underlying conditions and factors that can contribute to the development of CKD. Some of the primary causes include:

Diabetes: Diabetes is the leading cause of CKD worldwide. High blood sugar levels associated with diabetes can damage the blood vessels in the kidneys, impairing their ability to filter waste products effectively. Both type 1 and type 2 diabetes can lead to CKD, with the risk increasing as blood sugar levels remain poorly controlled.

Hypertension (high blood pressure): Hypertension is another significant cause of CKD. Elevated blood pressure can damage the blood vessels in the kidneys and reduce their ability to filter waste products properly. Over time, uncontrolled hypertension can lead to kidney damage and, eventually, kidney failure.

Glomerulonephritis: Glomerulonephritis is an inflammation of the glomeruli, the tiny filtering units within the kidneys. It can be caused by various factors, including infections, autoimmune diseases, or exposure to certain medications or toxins. Glomerulonephritis can lead to CKD if left untreated.

Polycystic kidney disease (PKD): PKD is a genetic disorder characterized by the growth of numerous cysts in the kidneys. These cysts can gradually enlarge and damage kidney tissue, leading to CKD.

Urinary tract obstructions: Blockages in the urinary tract, such as kidney stones, tumors, or an enlarged prostate, can obstruct the flow of urine and cause pressure buildup in the kidneys. Over time, this pressure can damage the kidneys and contribute to the development of CKD.

Risk Factors for CKD

Several risk factors can increase an individual's likelihood of developing CKD. Some of the primary risk factors include:

Age: The risk of developing CKD increases with age, particularly after 60 years. This is partly due to the natural decline in kidney function as we age and the increased prevalence of other risk factors, such as hypertension and diabetes, among older adults.

Family history: Having a family history of kidney disease, particularly a first-degree relative (parent or sibling), increases the risk of developing CKD.

Ethnicity: Certain ethnic groups, including African Americans, Hispanics, Native Americans, and Asians, have a higher prevalence of CKD compared to other populations. This increased risk is partly due to higher rates of diabetes and hypertension within these communities.

Obesity: Obesity is a significant risk factor for CKD, as it can contribute to the development of diabetes, hypertension, and other conditions that damage the kidneys.

Smoking: Smoking can damage blood vessels and decrease blood flow to the kidneys, increasing the risk of CKD. Additionally, smoking is associated with an increased risk of hypertension, another significant contributor to kidney damage.

Chronic use of certain medications: Long-term use of some medications, such as nonsteroidal anti-inflammatory drugs (NSAIDs) and certain antibiotics, can harm the kidneys and increase the risk of CKD.

Prevention and Management of CKD Risk Factors

By addressing these risk factors, individuals can significantly reduce their risk of developing CKD or slow its progression if already diagnosed. Key strategies for managing risk factors include:

Managing diabetes and hypertension: Regularly monitoring blood sugar and blood pressure levels, taking prescribed medications as directed, and making lifestyle modifications can help prevent or manage these conditions and their impact on kidney health.

Maintaining a healthy weight: Adopting a balanced diet and engaging in regular physical activity can help prevent obesity and its associated health risks, including CKD.

Quitting smoking: Smoking cessation is crucial for preserving kidney health and preventing CKD, as well as for reducing the risk of many other health problems. Consult a healthcare professional for support and resources to quit smoking.

Limiting the use of certain medications: Avoid long-term use of medications that can damage the kidneys, such as NSAIDs, and speak with a healthcare professional about safer alternatives when necessary. Always take medications as prescribed and discuss any concerns with a healthcare provider.

Regular check-ups: Regular health check-ups and screenings, particularly for those with risk factors, can help detect early signs of CKD and enable timely intervention to prevent or slow its progression.

Adopting a heart-healthy diet: Consuming a diet rich in fruits, vegetables, whole grains, lean proteins, and low-fat dairy can help manage blood pressure, blood sugar levels, and weight, which are essential factors in preserving kidney health. Limiting sodium, added sugars, and unhealthy fats is also crucial.

Staying hydrated: Drinking adequate water daily can help maintain proper kidney function and flush out waste products from the body. Be sure to consult a healthcare professional for specific recommendations based on individual needs and health status.

Understanding the causes and risk factors associated with CKD is essential for prevention and effective management of the disease. By adopting a healthy lifestyle and addressing modifiable risk factors, individuals can significantly reduce their risk of developing CKD and slow its progression if already diagnosed. Early detection and timely intervention are crucial to preserving kidney health and preventing the potentially severe complications associated with CKD.

HEART DISEASE IN CKD PATIENTS

Heart disease, also known as cardiovascular disease, is a major risk factor for individuals with chronic kidney disease (CKD). In fact, people with CKD are more likely to develop heart disease than those without kidney issues. This chapter aims to provide an overview of heart disease, common heart-related problems, and practical tips to reduce the risk of developing heart disease, with a special focus on aortic atherosclerosis.

Dr. Steven Rosansky, a nephrologist and the author of **Learn The Facts About Kidney Disease**, has discussed the relationship between heart disease and CKD extensively. As a regular co-host on Dadvice TV, he emphasizes the importance of understanding and managing heart disease for individuals with CKD.

Heart disease refers to a group of conditions that affect the heart and blood vessels. Some common heart-related issues include coronary artery disease, heart failure, arrhythmias, and valvular heart disease. Aortic atherosclerosis, which is the hardening and narrowing of the aorta due to the buildup of plaque, can be particularly dangerous for CKD patients.

A study by Matsushita et al. (2010) found that people with CKD had a higher prevalence of aortic atherosclerosis than those without CKD. This is alarming, as aortic atherosclerosis can lead to serious complications, such as heart attack, stroke, and even death.

Dr. Rosansky highlights several key strategies for CKD patients to reduce their risk of heart disease:

1. Control blood pressure: Maintaining a healthy blood pressure is crucial, as high blood pressure can damage both the heart and kidneys. Aim for a target blood pressure of 120/80 mm Hg or lower.
2. Manage diabetes: Diabetes is a major risk factor for heart disease. Work with your healthcare team to maintain proper blood sugar levels.
3. Maintain a healthy weight: Excess weight can strain the heart and increase the risk of heart disease. Aim for a body mass index (BMI) within the normal range.
4. Eat a heart-healthy diet: A diet low in saturated fats, trans fats, and cholesterol, and rich in fruits, vegetables, whole grains, lean proteins, and healthy fats can help reduce the risk of heart disease.
5. Be physically active: Regular exercise can improve heart health, lower blood pressure, and maintain a healthy weight. Aim for at least 150 minutes of moderate-intensity aerobic activity per week (30 minutes, 5 times a week for example).
6. Quit smoking: Smoking damages the heart and blood vessels, increasing the risk of heart disease. Quitting smoking is one of the best ways to improve heart health.
7. Limit alcohol consumption: Excessive alcohol intake can raise blood pressure and harm the heart. Stick to the recommended limits of no more than one drink per day for women and two drinks per day for men.
8. Manage stress: Chronic stress can contribute to heart disease. Practice stress-reducing techniques such as deep breathing, meditation, or yoga.

By following these tips and working closely with their healthcare team, individuals with CKD can take steps to prevent heart disease and improve their overall health. It is essential to take action and make lifestyle changes to protect the heart and reduce the risk of serious complications related to aortic atherosclerosis and other heart conditions.

Reference:

Matsushita, K., van der Velde, M., Astor, B. C., Woodward, M., Levey, A. S., de Jong, P. E., ... & Chronic Kidney Disease Prognosis Consortium. (2010). Association of estimated glomerular filtration rate and albuminuria with all-cause and cardiovascular mortality: a collaborative meta-analysis of general population cohorts. The Lancet, 375(9731), 2073-2081.

COLLABORATING WITH KIDNEY PROFESSIONALS

Navigating the world of kidney disease can be challenging, but collaborating with a team of kidney professionals is crucial for managing your condition effectively. This chapter will provide an overview of the various kidney professionals you may encounter, as well as tips for effectively communicating and building cooperative relationships with them.

A Comprehensive List of Kidney Professionals

Nephrologist: A nephrologist is a physician who specializes in the diagnosis, treatment, and management of kidney diseases. They will be your primary kidney specialist and play a crucial role in your care.

Primary Care Physician (PCP): Your PCP is responsible for managing your overall health and coordinating care with other specialists, like your nephrologist. They can help ensure that your treatment plan is consistent and addresses all aspects of your health.

Renal Dietitian: A renal dietitian is an expert in nutrition for kidney disease patients. They will work with you to create a customized meal plan that supports your kidney health and addresses any specific dietary needs or restrictions.

Social Worker: A social worker can provide support for the emotional and psychological aspects of living with kidney disease, as well as help you navigate the healthcare system, access resources, and address financial concerns.

Dialysis Technician: Dialysis technicians are trained professionals who assist with the dialysis process, ensuring that the equipment is functioning properly and providing care and support during your treatments.

Pharmacist: A pharmacist can help you manage your medications, provide information about potential side effects and drug interactions, and offer guidance on how to take your medications properly.

Transplant Coordinator: A transplant coordinator is a healthcare professional who helps manage the organ transplant process, from initial evaluation to post-transplant care. They serve as a liaison between you, your healthcare team, and the transplant center.

Tips for Effectively Communicating with Kidney Professionals

Be Prepared: Before your appointments, make a list of questions or concerns you have. Bring any relevant medical records, lab results, or medication lists to help your healthcare team better understand your situation.

Be Honest: Openly share your symptoms, concerns, and any challenges you may be facing. Your healthcare team can provide the best support and guidance when they have a clear understanding of your needs.

Ask Questions: Don't hesitate to ask for clarification or further explanation if you don't understand something. Remember that your healthcare team is there to help you.

Keep a Health Journal: Maintain a record of your symptoms, medications, and any changes in your health. This can help your healthcare team identify patterns and make informed decisions about your care.

Designate a Primary Decision Maker: Choose one healthcare professional, such as your PCP, to be the primary decision maker and coordinator of your care. This can help streamline communication and prevent confusion.

Building a Cooperative Relationship with Your Kidney Professionals

Establish Trust: Building trust with your healthcare team is essential for a successful collaboration. Be open and honest with them, and trust their expertise and guidance.

Stay Engaged: Actively participate in your care by asking questions, sharing your thoughts, and following your healthcare team's recommendations.

Be Patient: Building a strong relationship with your healthcare team takes time. Be patient, and recognize that your healthcare team is working towards your best interests.

Be Proactive: Take ownership of your health by educating yourself about kidney disease, following your treatment plan, and staying up-to-date on the latest research and recommendations.

Maintain Open Communication: Keep the lines of communication open with your healthcare team. Update them on any changes in your health or circumstances, and let them know if you are struggling with any aspects of your care.

Working with a Renal Dietitian

Working with a renal dietitian is a vital step in managing your kidney health. These specialized professionals are dedicated to helping kidney patients adopt a heart-healthy, kidney-friendly diet tailored to their individual needs. Their primary goal is to slow the progression of CKD and manage symptoms through proper nutrition.

When you begin working with a renal dietitian, the first visit typically involves a comprehensive assessment of your medical history, current diet, and lifestyle. They may ask about your preferences, allergies, and any specific dietary restrictions. Based on this information, the dietitian will develop a personalized meal plan that incorporates the right balance of nutrients, taking into account your kidney function and overall health.

Here are my top 7 benefits of working with a renal dietitian:

1. Personalized meal planning: A renal dietitian creates a customized meal plan tailored to your specific needs, taking into account your kidney function, medical history, and individual preferences.

2. Improved nutritional knowledge: Working with a renal dietitian helps you understand the impact of various nutrients on your kidney health and overall well-being, enabling you to make informed choices about your diet.

3. Better symptom management: A renal dietitian can help you manage symptoms associated with CKD, such as fatigue, swelling, and high blood pressure, through targeted dietary recommendations.

4. Slowing CKD progression: By implementing a kidney-friendly diet under the guidance of a renal dietitian, you may slow down the progression of CKD and potentially reduce the risk of kidney failure.

5. Enhanced quality of life: A renal dietitian can recommend foods and meal plans that not only support kidney health but also boost your energy levels, improve digestion, and promote general well-being.

6. Support for co-existing conditions: Many CKD patients have other health conditions like diabetes

or heart disease. A renal dietitian can help you manage these co-existing conditions through appropriate dietary adjustments.

7. Ongoing guidance and motivation: Working with a renal dietitian provides you with continuous support, encouragement, and accountability, ensuring you stay on track with your kidney-friendly diet and make lasting, positive changes to your eating habits.

Renal dietitians are available both locally and online, offering flexibility and accessibility for patients seeking expert guidance. Virtual services like Plant-Powered Kidneys (https://www.plantpoweredkidneys.com/) and the Kidney Nutrition Institute (https://kidneynutritioninstitute.org/) enable you to connect with professionals from the comfort of your home, making it even easier to access support on your journey towards better kidney health. By working with a renal dietitian, you empower yourself with knowledge and tools to make informed dietary choices and take control of your CKD management.

Coordinating Care Among Kidney Professionals

Handling care coordination among various kidney professionals can seem like a daunting task, but it's crucial for ensuring those with CKD receive all-encompassing, synchronized care. Here are some pointers for successfully managing care among kidney professionals:

1. Designate a central contact: Select a primary contact within your healthcare team, like your primary care physician, who can help orchestrate care among other kidney professionals.

2. Organize records diligently: Keep a well-structured system for storing medical records, lab results, and other relevant documents. This will simplify sharing information with various kidney

professionals and make sure everyone stays in the loop regarding CKD care.

3. **Adopt a shared care strategy:** Collaborate with the healthcare team to devise a shared care strategy that clarifies the roles and responsibilities of each kidney professional, as well as the objectives and tactics for CKD care. This can help streamline communication and coordination among kidney professionals.

4. **Hold routine check-ins:** Arrange regular check-ins with each kidney professional to discuss progress, tackle any concerns, and verify that everyone agrees on the CKD care strategy. These check-ins can happen in person, by phone, or through virtual appointments, based on individual preferences and the availability of kidney professionals.

5. **Embrace technology:** Use technology, like electronic health records and secure messaging platforms, to enable communication and coordination among kidney professionals. These tools can assist in keeping everyone informed and actively involved in the CKD care process.

6. **Take the initiative to overcome obstacles:** If any barriers to coordinating care among kidney professionals arise, such as scheduling conflicts or issues accessing medical records, confront them head-on and collaborate with the healthcare team to find solutions.

Collaborating with kidney professionals is an essential part of managing kidney disease and maintaining your overall health. By building strong relationships, staying engaged in your care, and effectively communicating with your healthcare team, you can ensure that you receive the best possible support and guidance on your kidney health journey. Remember that you are not alone, and your team of kidney professionals is there to help you navigate the challenges and complexities of living with kidney disease.

YOUR FIRST KIDNEY DOCTOR VISIT

Navigating your first appointment with a nephrologist can be an emotional rollercoaster, but being well-prepared can help alleviate some of the anxiety. To ensure a smooth experience, we've provided a step-by-step guide to help you navigate your first visit.

Take a deep breath and remember that it's okay to feel overwhelmed initially. Break down the preparation process into smaller tasks to avoid feeling swamped. Before your appointment, consider inviting a trusted friend or family member to join you for moral support and assistance with decision-making. In a dedicated notebook, write down any questions and concerns you'd like to address, and make sure to clarify the following details before your visit:

- The nature of the physical examination(s)
- Appropriate clothing for the appointment
- Whether a urine sample is needed upon arrival
- Parking instructions for the office or department

Aim to arrive 15 minutes early for your appointment, and ensure you have the following items and information on hand. Although not all of this will be shared directly with the doctor, it may be required by the registration clerk, medical assistant, or nurse:

- A list detailing your symptoms and their durations

- Contact information for all your current doctors
- An up-to-date list of medications
- Your insurance card
- A comprehensive medical history
- A record of past surgeries or medical procedures

Should you have additional resources, such as external lab work, let the office know during your appointment. If you're in the habit of tracking your blood pressure at home, bring along your blood pressure cuff for verification and review of your readings. Additionally, if you monitor your weight at home, provide a few recent records.

Questions to Ask Your Doctor

Upon being diagnosed with CKD, it's normal to feel overwhelmed during your doctor's appointments, as there is a plethora of information to process. One of the most effective ways to regain control and manage your condition is to become your own advocate. Don't hesitate to ask questions, seek clarification, or request repetition of information. If you find it challenging to be assertive, consider bringing a friend or family member along for support. Take notes during your appointments, as this will help you remember any additional questions or concerns that arise between visits. Embracing a proactive approach is essential when navigating the complexities of kidney disease. To help you get started, here are seven crucial questions to ask your doctor:

- What caused my kidney disease?
- What is my current stage of kidney disease and what does that mean?
- Can you explain my lab test results, including my glomerular filtration rate (eGFR)?
- What treatment options are available for my

specific symptoms?
- What are the next steps in managing my kidney disease?
- What actions can I take to prevent further damage to my kidneys?
- Will I eventually require dialysis or a kidney transplant, and if so, what is the expected timeline?

Asking these questions will not only provide you with valuable insights but also foster a more empathetic and collaborative relationship with your healthcare team. Remember, you have the power to take charge of your kidney health, and being well-informed is the first step.

UNDERSTANDING LABS AND DIAGNOSTICS

Regular monitoring of kidney function and associated markers is essential for individuals with chronic kidney disease (CKD). Proper interpretation of laboratory tests and diagnostic tools can help identify the progression of the disease, evaluate the effectiveness of treatments, and detect potential complications. This chapter will discuss the key laboratory tests and diagnostic tools used in the assessment and management of CKD, as well as the importance of understanding these results for optimal disease management.

Blood Tests

Several blood tests are used to monitor kidney function, detect potential complications, and assess overall health in individuals with CKD. These tests include:

1. Estimated glomerular filtration rate (eGFR): The eGFR is a measure of kidney function and is calculated using a blood test for creatinine, a waste product that is removed from the blood by the kidneys. The eGFR is expressed in milliliters per minute per 1.73 square meters (mL/min/1.73 m^2) and is adjusted for age, sex, and race. An eGFR below 60 for three months or more indicates CKD. The eGFR is used to classify CKD into five stages, with

lower values indicating more advanced disease.

2. Blood urea nitrogen (BUN): BUN is another waste product that is removed from the blood by the kidneys. Elevated BUN levels may indicate reduced kidney function, dehydration, or other factors that can affect kidney function.

3. Complete blood count (CBC): The CBC provides information about the number and types of cells in the blood, including red blood cells, white blood cells, and platelets. This test is used to assess overall health, detect anemia (a common complication of CKD), and monitor the response to treatments for anemia.

4. Electrolytes: The kidneys play a crucial role in maintaining the balance of electrolytes in the body, such as sodium, potassium, calcium, and phosphorus. Blood tests for electrolytes can help identify imbalances that may be indicative of CKD or potential complications, such as hyperkalemia (high potassium levels) or hyperphosphatemia (high phosphorus levels).

5. Parathyroid hormone (PTH): PTH is a hormone that helps regulate calcium and phosphorus levels in the body. Elevated PTH levels can be a sign of bone and mineral disorders in individuals with CKD, as the kidneys may struggle to maintain the balance of these minerals.

6. Albumin: Albumin is a protein found in the blood that helps maintain fluid balance and transport substances throughout the body. Low albumin levels may be a sign of malnutrition or inflammation in individuals with CKD.

Urine Tests

Urine tests are used to assess kidney function, detect potential complications, and evaluate the effectiveness of treatments for CKD. These tests include:

1. Urinalysis: A urinalysis involves a physical, chemical, and microscopic examination of a urine sample. This test can help detect abnormalities in the urine, such as the presence of blood (hematuria), excess protein (proteinuria), or signs of infection.

2. Urine albumin-to-creatinine ratio (UACR): The UACR is a measure of the amount of albumin (a protein) in the urine, which can be an early indicator of kidney damage. A UACR of 30 mg/g or higher is considered abnormal and may indicate CKD.

3. 24-hour urine collection: A 24-hour urine collection involves collecting all urine produced over a 24-hour period to measure the total volume of urine and assess the levels of various substances, such as protein or creatinine. This test can provide more accurate information about kidney function and help detect potential complications in individuals with CKD.

Imaging Studies

Imaging studies can be used to evaluate the size, shape, and structure of the kidneys, detect potential complications, or identify the underlying cause of CKD. These studies include:

1. Ultrasound: An ultrasound is a non-invasive imaging technique that uses sound waves to create images of the kidneys. This test can help detect structural abnormalities, such as kidney stones, cysts, or tumors, as well as assess blood flow to the kidneys.

2. Computed tomography (CT) scan: A CT scan is an imaging technique that uses X-rays and a computer to create detailed, cross-sectional images of the kidneys. This test can help detect structural abnormalities, such as kidney stones, cysts, or tumors, as well as assess blood flow to the kidneys. A CT scan may be performed with or without contrast, depending on the clinical situation and the individual's risk factors.

3. Magnetic resonance imaging (MRI): An MRI is an imaging technique that uses a magnetic field and radio waves to create detailed, cross-sectional images of the kidneys. This test can help detect structural abnormalities, such as kidney stones, cysts, or tumors, as well as assess blood flow to the kidneys. An MRI may be performed with or without contrast, depending on the clinical situation and the individual's risk factors.

Kidney Biopsy

A kidney biopsy is a medical procedure that involves obtaining a small sample of kidney tissue for examination under a microscope. This is typically done to diagnose kidney disease, determine the severity of the condition, or evaluate how well a treatment plan is working. During a kidney biopsy, a needle is inserted through the skin and into the kidney to collect the tissue sample. The procedure is usually performed under local anesthesia and may involve the use of ultrasound or other imaging techniques to help guide the needle to the appropriate location. The collected tissue is then analyzed by a pathologist to provide valuable information about the health and function of the kidneys.

IMPORTANT LAB TEST VALUES

As a kidney patient, it is crucial to familiarize yourself with the essential lab tests that monitor your kidney function and overall health. By understanding these tests and their normal ranges, you will be better equipped to track your progress, communicate with your healthcare team, and make informed decisions about your treatment plan. In this chapter, we will cover some of the most important lab tests for kidney patients, discuss their normal ranges, and explain what each test measures.

Albumin

Normal Range: 3.4-5.4 g/dL

Albumin is a protein made by the liver that helps maintain fluid balance and transports various substances through the bloodstream. Low albumin levels can indicate malnutrition or inflammation, both of which are common in kidney disease. Ensuring proper protein intake and managing inflammation can help maintain healthy albumin levels.

Blood Urea Nitrogen (BUN)

Normal Range: 7-20 mg/dL

BUN measures the amount of nitrogen in your blood that comes from the waste product urea, which is created when your body breaks down proteins. High BUN levels can indicate reduced kidney function, as the kidneys are less able to remove urea from the bloodstream. Treatment may involve adjusting protein intake, managing other health conditions, or altering medications.

Calcium

Normal Range: 8.6-10.2 mg/dL

Calcium is essential for strong bones, blood clotting, and proper nerve and muscle function. Kidney patients often experience imbalances in calcium levels, which can lead to bone disease, heart problems, or other complications. Treatment may involve dietary changes, medications, or dialysis adjustments.

Creatinine

Normal Range: Males - 0.74-1.35 mg/dL; Females - 0.59-1.04 mg/dL

Creatinine is a waste product that comes from the normal wear and tear on muscles in the body. High creatinine levels can indicate reduced kidney function, as the kidneys are less able to filter creatinine from the blood. Treatment may involve managing underlying health conditions, medications, or adjusting dialysis if applicable.

Estimated Glomerular Filtration Rate (eGFR)

Normal Range: >90 mL/min/1.73 m^2

eGFR is a calculation based on your creatinine level, age, sex, and race that estimates how well your kidneys are filtering waste from your blood. Lower eGFR values can indicate worsening kidney function, and treatment may involve managing underlying health conditions, medications, or dialysis if necessary. Your eGFR is NOT a static number and can fluctuate throughout the day, so focus on the trend and not a single value. It is natural for your eGFR to decline by approximately 1 point each year after 40.

Hematocrit (HCT)

Normal Range: Males - 38.8-50%; Females - 34.9-44.5%

Hematocrit measures the proportion of red blood cells in

your blood. A low HCT can indicate anemia, a common complication in kidney disease, as the kidneys produce less of the hormone erythropoietin, which stimulates red blood cell production. Treating anemia may involve iron supplementation, erythropoiesis-stimulating agents, or blood transfusions.

Hemoglobin

Normal Range: Males - 13.5-17.5 g/dL; Females: 12.0-15.5 g/dL

Hemoglobin is an essential component of red blood cells that carries oxygen from your lungs to the rest of your body. Low hemoglobin levels (anemia) are common in kidney disease, as the kidneys produce a hormone called erythropoietin, which stimulates red blood cell production. Anemia can cause fatigue, weakness, and shortness of breath.

A1c (A1c)

Normal Range: 4-5.6%

The A1c test measures your average blood sugar levels over the past 2-3 months. High A1c levels can indicate poor blood sugar control in people with diabetes, a major risk factor for kidney disease. Maintaining proper blood sugar control is essential for preventing or managing kidney damage in diabetic patients.

High-Density Lipoprotein (HDL)

Normal Range: Males - >40 mg/dL; Females - >50 mg/dL

HDL cholesterol is often called "good" cholesterol because it helps remove harmful cholesterol from the bloodstream, reducing the risk of heart disease. Higher levels of HDL are generally considered better for heart health.

Low-Density Lipoprotein (LDL)

Normal Range: <100 mg/dL

LDL cholesterol is often called "bad" cholesterol because it contributes to the buildup of plaque in the arteries, increasing the risk of heart disease. Lowering LDL levels can be achieved through lifestyle changes and medications, if necessary.

Phosphorus

Normal Range: 2.5-4.5 mg/dL

Phosphorus is a mineral that works with calcium to help build strong bones and teeth. In kidney disease, the kidneys may have difficulty removing excess phosphorus from the blood, leading to high levels that can cause bone and heart problems. Managing phosphorus levels may involve dietary changes, phosphate binders, or adjustments to dialysis.

Potassium

Normal Range: 3.5-5.0 mEq/L

Potassium is an essential mineral that helps maintain proper nerve and muscle function, including the heart. In kidney disease, the kidneys may struggle to maintain normal potassium levels, leading to imbalances that can cause irregular heartbeats or other complications. Treatment may involve dietary changes, medications, or dialysis adjustments.

Red Blood Cells (RBC)

Normal Range: Males - 4.7-6.1 million cells/mcL; Females - 4.2-5.4 million cells/mcL

Red blood cells carry oxygen from the lungs to the rest of the body and remove carbon dioxide. A low RBC count can indicate anemia, a common complication in kidney disease. Treatment for anemia may involve iron supplementation, erythropoiesis-stimulating agents, or blood transfusions.

Sodium

Normal Range: 135-145 mEq/L

Sodium is an essential electrolyte that helps maintain fluid balance and proper nerve and muscle function. Imbalances in sodium levels can occur in kidney disease, leading to complications such as high blood pressure or fluid retention. Treatment may involve dietary changes, medications, or dialysis adjustments.

Total Cholesterol (TC)

Normal Range: <200 mg/dL

Total cholesterol is a measure of the cholesterol in your blood, including both "good" (HDL) and "bad" (LDL) cholesterol. High total cholesterol levels can increase the risk of heart disease, and managing cholesterol levels is important for overall cardiovascular health.

Triglycerides

Normal Range: <150 mg/dL

Triglycerides are a type of fat found in your blood that your body uses for energy. High triglyceride levels can increase the risk of heart disease. Lowering triglycerides may involve lifestyle changes, such as diet and exercise, or medications if necessary.

Uric Acid

Normal Range: Males - 3.4-7.0 mg/dL; Females - 2.4-6.0 mg/dL

Uric acid is a waste product that results from the breakdown of purines, which are found in certain foods and produced by the body. High uric acid levels can lead to gout or kidney stones and may be associated with reduced kidney function. Treatment may involve dietary changes, medications, or managing underlying health conditions.

Vitamin D

Normal Range: 20-50 ng/mL

Vitamin D is essential for maintaining strong bones and a healthy immune system. In kidney disease, the kidneys may struggle to activate vitamin D, leading to low levels that can contribute to bone disease or other complications. Treatment may involve vitamin D supplementation, managing phosphorus and calcium levels, or adjusting dialysis if applicable.

Understanding and keeping track of these lab tests and their values is crucial for kidney patients. By staying informed about your test results, you can work closely with your healthcare team to make the best decisions regarding your treatment plan and lifestyle adjustments. Remember, knowledge is power, and being proactive in managing your kidney health can significantly improve your quality of life and outcomes.

Leveraging Lab Results to Guide Informed Decisions

As a kidney patient, I've found that using my lab results to prepare questions for my doctor has been instrumental in making better diet and lifestyle decisions. When my lab results are posted on the patient website or app, I carefully review them to identify any values that fall outside the normal range.

For each of these values, I create a list of questions to ask my doctor, focusing on the potential causes and the steps I can take to bring the values within the normal range. This approach allows me to better understand the factors affecting my kidney health and empowers me to take proactive steps to address them.

Once I've compiled my list of questions, I email them to my doctor in advance of our next appointment, giving them enough time to review and prepare answers. This not only ensures a more efficient use of our time together but also allows for a more in-depth discussion of my concerns.

During the appointment, we go through each question, and my doctor provides guidance on what I can do to improve my lab values. By following this method, I've been able to get nearly all of my lab values within the normal range over time, significantly enhancing my kidney health and overall well-being.

EGFR AND PROTEIN LEAKAGE

Understanding the relationship between eGFR and protein leakage is essential for individuals with chronic kidney disease (CKD). This chapter will discuss the significance of eGFR and protein leakage, their connection, and the importance of monitoring these two factors in the management of CKD.

Estimated Glomerular Filtration Rate (eGFR)

eGFR, or estimated glomerular filtration rate, is a measure of kidney function calculated using a blood test for creatinine, a waste product removed from the blood by the kidneys. The eGFR is expressed in milliliters per minute per 1.73 square meters (mL/min/1.73 m2) and is adjusted for age, sex, and race. It's essential to understand that eGFR is a snapshot in time and can fluctuate throughout the day, so it's not a fixed number. In fact, eGFR is more like a small range than a single value. However, eGFR may not be entirely accurate for certain individuals, such as those younger than 18, pregnant, very overweight, or very muscular. In these cases, healthcare professionals may need to consider additional factors or tests to assess kidney function accurately.

Factors that affect eGFR

Several factors can influence eGFR, including:

- Age: Kidney function naturally declines with age, which can result in lower eGFR values in older individuals.

- Sex: eGFR values are typically lower in women compared to men, due to differences in muscle mass and creatinine production.
- Race: eGFR values may differ among racial and ethnic groups, with African Americans and certain other groups typically having higher eGFR values compared to Caucasians.
- Medications: Some medications can affect eGFR by influencing creatinine levels or kidney function.
- Medical conditions: Conditions such as diabetes, hypertension, or heart disease can impact eGFR by causing damage to the kidneys or altering kidney function.

It is essential to consider these factors when interpreting eGFR results and to discuss any concerns with a healthcare provider.

Tracking Your eGFR

Monitoring your eGFR is an essential aspect of managing your kidney health, as it provides valuable insights into your kidney function. However, it's crucial to remember that eGFR can fluctuate throughout the day, so small changes in the value should not be a cause for concern.

When tracking your eGFR, it's more important to focus on the overall trends rather than individual values. Observing these trends can help you and your healthcare team identify any significant changes in your kidney function and adjust your treatment plan accordingly.

To effectively track your eGFR, consider the following tips:

1. Keep a record: Maintain a log of your eGFR values, including the date of each test, to help you visualize the trends over time. This can be done using a notebook, spreadsheet, or a dedicated app.

2. Don't panic over small changes: Minor fluctuations in eGFR are normal and should not cause alarm. Keep in mind that eGFR is more of a range than a precise value.
3. Look for patterns: Analyze the data for any patterns or trends that may indicate improvements or declines in your kidney function. Share this information with your healthcare team to help them make informed decisions about your care.
4. Stay consistent: Try to schedule your blood tests at similar times of the day and under similar conditions to minimize the impact of daily fluctuations on your eGFR results.

Protein Leakage

Protein leakage, also known as proteinuria, is the presence of excess protein in the urine. The kidneys typically filter out waste products while retaining essential proteins in the bloodstream. However, when the kidneys are damaged, they may allow proteins, such as albumin, to pass through the filtration barrier and enter the urine.

Protein leakage is not only a symptom of kidney damage but also a predictor of future problems. The more protein a person leaks in their urine, the more likely their kidney disease will progress. Proteinuria can also contribute to further kidney damage and increased cardiovascular risk.

Factors that affect protein leakage

Several factors can influence protein leakage, including:

- Medical conditions: Conditions such as diabetes, hypertension, or lupus can cause kidney damage and lead to protein leakage.
- Infections: Urinary tract infections, kidney

infections, or other systemic infections can temporarily increase protein leakage.

- Medications: Some medications can affect protein leakage by influencing kidney function or altering the filtration barrier.
- Strenuous exercise: Intense physical activity can temporarily increase protein leakage due to increased muscle breakdown and subsequent release of proteins into the bloodstream.
- Dehydration: Dehydration can concentrate the urine and result in higher protein levels in the urine.

It is essential to consider these factors when interpreting protein leakage results and to discuss any concerns with a healthcare provider.

The Connection Between eGFR and Protein Leakage

The relationship between eGFR and protein leakage is crucial in understanding the progression of CKD. As kidney function declines (indicated by a lower eGFR), the amount of protein leakage typically increases. This is because the damaged kidneys are less efficient at retaining essential proteins and filtering waste products.

Protein leakage can exacerbate kidney damage, further reducing eGFR and accelerating the progression of CKD. In turn, a declining eGFR can lead to an increase in protein leakage, creating a cycle of worsening kidney function.

REDUCING PROTEIN IN THE URINE

Proteinuria, or the presence of excessive protein in the urine, is a common indicator of kidney damage and a risk factor for the progression of chronic kidney disease (CKD). Reducing proteinuria is an essential aspect of managing kidney disease and slowing its progression. In this chapter, we will discuss the common medications and lifestyle tips that can help decrease protein in the urine.

Common Medications for Reducing Proteinuria

Angiotensin-converting enzyme inhibitors (ACE inhibitors) and angiotensin II receptor blockers (ARBs) are two classes of medications commonly prescribed to reduce proteinuria in individuals with kidney disease. These medications work by decreasing the pressure inside the glomeruli (the tiny blood vessels in the kidneys), which helps reduce protein leakage and protect the kidneys from further damage.

1. ACE Inhibitors: ACE inhibitors work by blocking the action of the enzyme responsible for the production of angiotensin II, a hormone that narrows blood vessels and increases blood pressure. Some common ACE inhibitors include:

   - Benazepril (Lotensin)
   - Captopril (Capoten)
   - Enalapril (Vasotec)

- Fosinopril (Monopril)
- Lisinopril (Prinivil, Zestril)
- Quinapril (Accupril)
- Ramipril (Altace)

2. ARBs: ARBs block the action of angiotensin II by preventing it from binding to its receptor. This helps relax blood vessels and lower blood pressure. Some common ARBs include:

- Candesartan (Atacand)
- Irbesartan (Avapro)
- Losartan (Cozaar)
- Olmesartan (Benicar)
- Telmisartan (Micardis)
- Valsartan (Diovan)

Your healthcare provider will determine the most appropriate medication for your situation based on your medical history, kidney function, and other factors. It's essential to take these medications as prescribed and report any side effects to your healthcare provider.

Lifestyle Tips for Reducing Proteinuria

In addition to medications, there are several lifestyle changes that can help reduce protein in the urine and improve kidney health:

1. Maintain a Healthy Blood Pressure: High blood pressure can contribute to kidney damage and proteinuria. Monitor your blood pressure regularly and follow your healthcare provider's recommendations for managing high blood pressure, such as taking prescribed medications, reducing sodium intake, and maintaining a healthy

weight.

2. Control Blood Sugar Levels: If you have diabetes, keeping your blood sugar levels in check is crucial for preventing kidney damage and reducing proteinuria. Work with your healthcare team to develop a diabetes management plan, including proper diet, exercise, and medications if necessary.

3. Follow a Kidney-Friendly Diet: A diet tailored to your specific needs can help reduce proteinuria and maintain kidney health. This may include limiting protein intake, controlling sodium and potassium levels, and avoiding high-phosphorus foods. Consult a renal dietitian for personalized guidance.

4. Stay Active: Regular physical activity can help manage blood pressure, blood sugar levels, and weight, all of which contribute to kidney health. Aim for at least 30 minutes of low-impact exercise five days a week, such as walking, cycling, or swimming.

5. Avoid Nonsteroidal Anti-Inflammatory Drugs (NSAIDs): NSAIDs, such as ibuprofen and naproxen, can harm kidney function and increase proteinuria. Talk to your healthcare provider about alternative pain relief options if you regularly take NSAIDs.

6. Quit Smoking: Smoking can increase blood pressure and harm kidney function, contributing to proteinuria. If you smoke, work with your healthcare provider to develop a plan to quit.

By combining medication management with lifestyle changes, you can effectively reduce proteinuria and protect your kidneys from further damage. It's important to work closely with your healthcare team to monitor your progress and make adjustments as needed to optimize kidney health.

1. Maintain a Healthy Weight: Excess weight can contribute to high blood pressure and strain your kidneys. Work with your healthcare team to determine an appropriate weight for your height and body type, and develop a plan to achieve and maintain that weight through a balanced diet and regular exercise.

2. Manage Stress: Chronic stress can negatively impact your overall health and well-being, including your kidney health. Find healthy ways to cope with stress, such as practicing mindfulness, deep breathing exercises, or engaging in hobbies that bring you joy and relaxation.

3. Stay Hydrated: Drinking enough water is essential for maintaining healthy kidney function. While the optimal amount of water intake can vary depending on your specific kidney function and overall health, generally aim for at least eight 8-ounce glasses of water per day. Talk to your healthcare provider to determine the appropriate amount of fluid intake for your situation.

4. Regular Check-ups and Monitoring: Stay in close communication with your healthcare team and attend regular check-ups to monitor your kidney function, proteinuria levels, and overall health. This will help you identify any changes in your condition and adjust your treatment plan accordingly.

By implementing these lifestyle changes and working closely with your healthcare team, you can effectively reduce proteinuria, preserve kidney function, and slow the progression of chronic kidney disease. Remember, early intervention and consistent management are crucial for achieving the best possible outcomes in kidney disease.

LIVING WITH CHRONIC KIDNEY DISEASE

Coping with chronic kidney disease (CKD) can be demanding, but with the proper knowledge, support, and strategies, it's possible to maintain a good quality of life while managing the condition. This chapter will delve into various aspects of living with CKD, providing guidance on tackling the physical, emotional, and practical challenges that may arise.

Adapting to Daily Life with CKD

Establishing Routines: Creating a consistent routine for managing CKD can help individuals gain a sense of control over their condition. This may involve setting regular times for taking medications, attending medical appointments, exercising, and preparing meals.

Time Management: Living with CKD may necessitate additional time for self-care activities, such as meal preparation, exercise, and medical appointments. By prioritizing tasks and organizing time efficiently, individuals can ensure they have adequate time to care for their kidney health while still participating in work, hobbies, and social activities.

Managing Fatigue: Fatigue is a common CKD symptom that can significantly impact daily life. To manage fatigue, prioritize rest, maintain a consistent sleep schedule, and practice good sleep hygiene. Additionally, engaging in regular physical activity and managing stress can help improve energy levels.

Navigating the Healthcare System

Building a Healthcare Team: Collaborating with a multidisciplinary healthcare team is essential for managing CKD. This team may include a nephrologist, primary care physician, dietitian, pharmacist, and mental health professional. By cultivating a strong relationship with these providers, individuals can ensure they receive comprehensive care tailored to their needs.

Communicating with Healthcare Providers: Transparent and honest communication with healthcare providers is crucial for effective CKD management. Individuals should feel at ease discussing their symptoms, concerns, and treatment goals with their healthcare team and asking questions about their care.

Managing Medical Appointments: Regular medical appointments are necessary for monitoring CKD progression and adjusting treatments as needed. To maximize these appointments, individuals should come prepared with a list of questions, concerns, and any recent changes in their health.

Emotional Well-being and Support

Coping with Emotions: Living with CKD can evoke various emotions, including fear, sadness, anger, and frustration. Developing healthy coping strategies, such as journaling, practicing mindfulness, or engaging in creative outlets, can help individuals process these emotions and maintain emotional well-being.

Building a Support Network: A robust support network is vital for managing CKD's emotional challenges. This network may include family, friends, healthcare providers, and support groups. By connecting with others who understand their experiences, individuals can find encouragement, empathy, and practical advice for living with CKD.

Employment and Finances

Working with CKD: Many individuals with CKD continue to work, while others may need to modify their job responsibilities or work hours to accommodate their health needs. It's essential to communicate with employers about any necessary accommodations and be aware of legal rights and protections, such as the Family and Medical Leave Act (FMLA) or the Americans with Disabilities Act (ADA). For me, I only had challenges working when my kidney function was below eGFR 13.

Financial Planning: CKD can have financial implications, such as increased medical expenses or changes in employment status. Developing a financial plan, including budgeting for medical costs and exploring insurance options, can help individuals navigate the financial challenges of living with CKD.

Social Life and Relationships

Maintaining Social Connections: Engaging in social activities and maintaining relationships with friends and family is essential for emotional well-being while living with CKD. By communicating openly about their health needs and seeking support from loved ones, individuals can continue to enjoy social connections and build a strong support network.

Navigating Romantic Relationships: CKD may impact romantic relationships, particularly when it comes to intimacy, communication, and caregiving roles. By fostering open and honest communication with partners about their experiences and needs, individuals can work together to maintain a strong and supportive relationship.

Participating in Social Activities: While living with CKD may require some adjustments to social activities, individuals can still enjoy many of their favorite pastimes. This may involve adapting activities to accommodate physical limitations or fatigue, or finding new hobbies that are compatible with their health needs.

Traveling with CKD

Preparing for Travel: Traveling with CKD may require careful planning and preparation to ensure health needs are met while away from home, especially for those with kidney failure. This may include discussing travel plans with healthcare providers, researching nearby medical facilities, and packing necessary medications and supplies. I continue to travel for work and pleasure without any issues, including internationally.

Managing Healthcare Needs During Travel: While traveling, individuals should continue to adhere to their treatment plan, including taking medications, monitoring blood pressure, and maintaining dietary restrictions. By staying vigilant about their health needs, individuals can enjoy their travels while minimizing potential risks to their kidney health.

Advocating for Kidney Health

Raising Awareness: By sharing their experiences with CKD and educating others about kidney health, individuals can help raise awareness about the importance of early detection and management of kidney disease.

Advocating for Policy Changes: Individuals can advocate for policies and initiatives that support kidney health, such as increased funding for research, improved access to care, and expanded insurance coverage for CKD treatments.

Living with chronic kidney disease presents various challenges, but with the right knowledge, support, and strategies in place, individuals can maintain a good quality of life while managing their condition. By focusing on various aspects of living with CKD, such as daily routines, healthcare management, emotional well-being, and social relationships, individuals can better cope with their condition and continue to enjoy a fulfilling life.

LIFESTYLE CHANGES TO SLOW CKD AND LIVE LONGER

Living with chronic kidney disease (CKD) can be challenging, but adopting specific lifestyle changes can help slow its progression and extend your life. In this chapter, we will discuss various lifestyle modifications that can contribute to living a longer and healthier life with CKD.

Adopt a Kidney-Friendly Diet: Following a diet specifically designed for kidney health is essential to slow down CKD progression. Collaborate with your healthcare team or dietitian to create a personalized meal plan that focuses on limiting sodium, phosphorus, and, if necessary, potassium and protein intake. Ensure that you consume an adequate amount of calories, vitamins, and minerals to maintain a healthy weight and support your immune system.

Manage Blood Pressure: High blood pressure is a significant risk factor for CKD progression. Keeping your blood pressure within a healthy range is crucial. Achieve this by adhering to a low-sodium diet, taking prescribed medications, engaging in regular physical activity, and managing stress.

Control Blood Sugar Levels: If you have diabetes, managing your blood sugar levels is critical in slowing CKD progression. Work with your healthcare team to develop a diabetes management plan that includes a tailored diet, medications, and regular blood sugar monitoring.

Stay Active: Regular exercise is essential for overall health, maintaining a healthy weight, managing blood pressure and blood sugar levels, and promoting mental well-being. Aim for at least 30 minutes of low-impact exercise, such as walking, swimming, or cycling, most days of the week. Consult your healthcare team before starting any new exercise regimen.

Maintain a Healthy Weight: Carrying excess weight can put additional strain on your kidneys and contribute to high blood pressure and diabetes, both of which can exacerbate CKD. Work with your healthcare team to determine a healthy weight for you and develop a plan to achieve and maintain it through diet and exercise.

Stop Smoking: Smoking is harmful to your kidneys and can accelerate CKD progression. Quitting smoking can significantly improve your kidney health and extend your life expectancy. Consider seeking support from smoking cessation programs or healthcare professionals to help you quit.

Limit Alcohol Consumption: Excessive alcohol intake can contribute to kidney damage and high blood pressure. To protect your kidneys and maintain overall health, either limit your alcohol consumption or abstain from it altogether.

Prioritize Sleep: Adequate sleep is essential for overall health and well-being. Aim for 7-8 hours of quality sleep each night. Establish a consistent sleep schedule, create a comfortable sleep environment, and practice good sleep hygiene to improve your sleep quality.

Manage Stress: Chronic stress can negatively impact your physical and mental health, making CKD management more difficult. Practice stress-reduction techniques like meditation, deep breathing exercises, yoga, or mindfulness to help alleviate stress and improve your quality of life.

Stay Informed and Educated: Staying up-to-date on the latest research and advancements in CKD treatment can empower you in managing your condition. Educate yourself to have more productive conversations with your healthcare team and play an active role in your treatment plan.

Build a Support Network: Connecting with others who share your experiences, such as support groups, online forums, or friends and family, can provide emotional support, practical advice, and encouragement. A strong support network can improve your quality of life and help you better manage your condition.

By focusing on these lifestyle changes and working closely with your healthcare team, you can take control of your CKD, slow its progression, and live a longer, healthier life.

MEDICATIONS AND SUPPLEMENTS FOR KIDNEY HEALTH

Effectively managing chronic kidney disease (CKD) often involves using medications and supplements to address various aspects of the condition, including blood pressure control, anemia management, and maintaining mineral balance. In this chapter, we delve into the common medications and supplements used in CKD management, exploring their benefits, potential side effects, and considerations for their use.

Blood pressure medications

Angiotensin-converting enzyme (ACE) inhibitors: ACE inhibitors, such as lisinopril, enalapril, and ramipril, function by relaxing blood vessels, lowering blood pressure, and reducing strain on the kidneys. They can slow the progression of CKD, particularly for individuals with diabetes.

Angiotensin II receptor blockers (ARBs): ARBs, including losartan, valsartan, and irbesartan, also help relax blood vessels and lower blood pressure. They serve as an alternative for individuals who cannot tolerate ACE inhibitors due to side effects such as a persistent cough.

Calcium channel blockers: These medications, such as amlodipine, nifedipine, and diltiazem, work by preventing calcium from entering heart and blood vessel cells, resulting in relaxed blood vessels and reduced blood pressure.

Beta-blockers: Beta-blockers like metoprolol, atenolol, and bisoprolol reduce blood pressure by blocking the effects of the hormone adrenaline, causing the heart to beat slower and with less force.

Anemia management

Erythropoiesis-stimulating agents (ESAs): ESAs, including epoetin alfa and darbepoetin alfa, stimulate red blood cell production in bone marrow, addressing anemia in individuals with CKD. These medications are typically administered via injection.

Iron supplements: Iron supplementation may be necessary for individuals with CKD-related anemia since iron is a crucial component of hemoglobin, the protein in red blood cells that carries oxygen. Iron supplements can be taken orally or administered intravenously, depending on individual needs and anemia severity.

Vitamin B12 and folic acid: These vitamins are vital for producing healthy red blood cells. Individuals with CKD may require supplementation, particularly if they take medications affecting the absorption or metabolism of these nutrients.

Mineral balance and bone health

Phosphate binders: High phosphorus levels in the blood can contribute to bone disease and cardiovascular complications in individuals with CKD. Phosphate binders like calcium carbonate, calcium acetate, and sevelamer are taken with meals to bind dietary phosphorus and reduce its absorption.

Vitamin D analogs: Vitamin D is crucial for maintaining bone health and regulating calcium and phosphorus levels. Individuals with CKD often have low active vitamin D levels due to decreased kidney function. Vitamin D analogs, such as calcitriol and paricalcitol, can be prescribed to help maintain proper mineral balance and promote bone health.

Calcimimetics: Calcimimetics like cinacalcet treat secondary hyperparathyroidism in individuals with advanced CKD. These medications mimic calcium's effects on the parathyroid glands, regulating parathyroid hormone release and maintaining proper calcium and phosphorus levels.

Diuretics

Loop diuretics: These medications, including furosemide, bumetanide, and torsemide, help kidneys remove excess fluid and sodium from the body by increasing urine production. Loop diuretics are commonly used in individuals with CKD to manage fluid overload and reduce swelling.

Thiazide diuretics: Thiazide diuretics, such as hydrochlorothiazide and chlorthalidone, also increase urine production to remove excess fluid and sodium. They may be used in combination with other blood pressure medications for individuals with CKD.

Potassium-sparing diuretics: Potassium-sparing diuretics, like spironolactone and eplerenone, help remove excess fluid while preserving potassium levels in the blood. They may be used in combination with other diuretics or blood pressure medications to prevent low potassium levels.

Cholesterol-lowering medications

Statins: Statins, such as atorvastatin, simvastatin, and rosuvastatin, are used to lower cholesterol levels, reducing the risk of heart disease and stroke in individuals with CKD. Statins work by inhibiting an enzyme involved in cholesterol production in the liver.

Ezetimibe: Ezetimibe is a cholesterol-absorption inhibitor that works by blocking cholesterol absorption from the small intestine. It may be used alone or in combination with statins to help lower cholesterol levels in individuals with CKD.

Blood sugar control

Insulin: Insulin is a hormone that regulates blood sugar levels. Individuals with diabetes and CKD may require insulin injections to maintain proper blood sugar control, as high blood sugar can contribute to kidney damage.

Oral diabetes medications: Several classes of oral diabetes medications, such as metformin, sulfonylureas, and DPP-4 inhibitors, can help manage blood sugar levels in individuals with diabetes and CKD. Healthcare providers will consider factors such as kidney function, potential side effects, and drug interactions when selecting appropriate medications.

Supplements and over-the-counter medications

Omega-3 fatty acids: Omega-3 fatty acid supplements, like fish oil, may offer anti-inflammatory and cardiovascular benefits for individuals with CKD. Discussing supplementation with a healthcare provider is recommended to determine the appropriate dosage and ensure there are no contraindications.

Probiotics: Probiotic supplements, which contain beneficial bacteria, may help improve gut health and reduce inflammation in individuals with CKD. However, more research is needed to determine their efficacy and safety in this population.

Over-the-counter medications: Some over-the-counter medications, such as nonsteroidal anti-inflammatory drugs (NSAIDs), can be harmful to kidney health. Individuals with CKD should consult with their healthcare provider before using any over-the-counter medications to ensure they are safe and appropriate for their condition.

Pain management

Acetaminophen: Acetaminophen, commonly known as Tylenol, is a relatively safe option for pain relief in individuals with CKD when used according to the recommended dosage. However, long-term use or exceeding the recommended dose can lead to liver damage. It is essential to consult with a healthcare provider before using acetaminophen for pain management.

Opioids: Opioids, such as morphine, oxycodone, and hydrocodone, can be used to manage moderate to severe pain in individuals with CKD. However, these medications have potential side effects, including drowsiness, constipation, and risk of dependence. Healthcare providers will carefully consider the risks and benefits before prescribing opioids for CKD patients.

Topical analgesics: Topical analgesics, such as lidocaine or capsaicin cream, can provide localized pain relief for individuals with CKD. These medications are applied directly to the skin over the affected area and may be a safer alternative to oral pain medications.

Managing gastrointestinal symptoms

Antacids: Antacids, such as aluminum hydroxide or magnesium hydroxide, can help neutralize stomach acid and provide relief from heartburn and indigestion. However, some antacids may interact with medications commonly prescribed for CKD, so individuals should consult with their healthcare provider before using antacids.

H2 blockers: H2 blockers, such as famotidine and ranitidine, reduce stomach acid production and can be used to manage heartburn, indigestion, and gastroesophageal reflux disease (GERD) in individuals with CKD. Healthcare providers will carefully consider the potential benefits and risks before prescribing these medications.

Proton pump inhibitors (PPIs): PPIs, such as omeprazole and pantoprazole, are another class of medications used to reduce stomach acid production. They may be prescribed for individuals with CKD who have GERD or other acid-related gastrointestinal issues. However, long-term use of PPIs has been associated with an increased risk of fractures and kidney disease, so their use should be carefully monitored.

Managing CKD often involves a combination of medications and supplements to address various aspects of the condition. It is crucial to work closely with a healthcare provider to develop a personalized treatment plan that considers individual needs, potential side effects, and drug interactions.

THE LATEST MEDICATIONS TO TREAT CKD

The landscape of CKD treatment has seen significant advancements in recent years, with innovative medications offering new options for patients. This chapter delves into the latest developments in CKD treatment and explores two of the most promising drug classes, SGLT-2 inhibitors and GLP-1 receptor agonists. By reviewing the latest research, we aim to provide a comprehensive understanding of these medications and their potential benefits for individuals living with CKD.

SGLT-2 Inhibitors

Sodium-glucose cotransporter-2 (SGLT-2) inhibitors have emerged as a groundbreaking treatment option for CKD patients, especially those with type 2 diabetes. These drugs work by blocking the reabsorption of glucose in the kidneys, allowing excess glucose to be excreted in the urine. This process helps lower blood sugar levels and has been shown to provide additional benefits such as blood pressure control and weight loss.

Recent research indicates that SGLT-2 inhibitors can also slow the progression of CKD. The groundbreaking DAPA-CKD trial published in The New England Journal of Medicine showed that dapagliflozin, an SGLT-2 inhibitor, reduced the risk of kidney function decline, end-stage kidney disease, and death from kidney or cardiovascular causes in patients with CKD and type 2 diabetes. Importantly, the study also demonstrated benefits for CKD patients without diabetes, suggesting that SGLT-2 inhibitors have potential as a treatment for a broader population. (Source: https://www.nejm.org/doi/full/10.1056/NEJMoa2024816)

SGLT-2 Inhibitors:

- Canagliflozin (Invokana)
- Dapagliflozin (Farxiga)
- Empagliflozin (Jardiance)
- Ertugliflozin (Steglatro)
- Sotagliflozin (Zynquista)

SGLT-2 inhibitors Drawbacks

SGLT-2 inhibitors, while effective in managing blood sugar levels in people with type 2 diabetes and showing benefits for kidney health, also come with some potential drawbacks and side effects. Some of the most common drawbacks of SGLT-2 inhibitors include:

Genital infections: SGLT-2 inhibitors can increase the risk of yeast infections in both men and women, as they increase glucose excretion in the urine, creating a favorable environment for fungal growth.

Urinary tract infections (UTIs): These medications may increase the risk of UTIs due to the increased glucose in the urine.

Dehydration: SGLT-2 inhibitors promote the excretion of glucose through the urine, which can also lead to fluid loss and dehydration, especially in elderly patients or those taking diuretics.

Hypotension: Dehydration and fluid loss can also lead to a drop in blood pressure, which may cause dizziness, lightheadedness, or fainting.

Ketoacidosis: Although rare, SGLT-2 inhibitors can increase the risk of diabetic ketoacidosis, a serious and life-threatening condition that occurs when the body produces high levels of blood acids called ketones.

Bone fractures: Some studies have suggested that SGLT-2 inhibitors may be linked to an increased risk of bone fractures due to factors such as dehydration, electrolyte imbalances, and a potential impact on bone density.

Amputations: Canagliflozin (Invokana) has been associated with an increased risk of lower limb amputations, although this risk has not been observed with other SGLT-2 inhibitors.

Drug interactions: SGLT-2 inhibitors may interact with other medications, such as diuretics, insulin, or other diabetes medications, which could lead to side effects or reduced effectiveness.

Cost of SGLT-2 inhibitors

The affordability of SGLT-2 inhibitors can vary depending on factors such as the specific medication, your location, your insurance coverage, and any available discounts or patient assistance programs. In general, SGLT-2 inhibitors can be quite expensive without insurance coverage or discounts.

Many insurance plans, including Medicare and Medicaid, do cover SGLT-2 inhibitors, but the extent of coverage may vary depending on the specific plan and medication. Some insurance plans may require prior authorization, step therapy, or impose quantity limits for these medications. It's essential to check with your insurance provider to understand the coverage for SGLT-2 inhibitors and any associated costs, such as copays or deductibles.

If you do not have insurance or your insurance does not provide adequate coverage for SGLT-2 inhibitors, there are other options to explore. Some pharmaceutical companies offer patient assistance programs or discount cards to help reduce the cost of these medications for eligible patients. Additionally, there are prescription discount services and generic versions of some SGLT-2 inhibitors that may help lower the cost. It is essential to discuss these options with your healthcare provider or pharmacist to find the most affordable solution for your situation.

It is essential to discuss these potential drawbacks and side effects with your healthcare provider before starting an SGLT-2 inhibitor to ensure the medication is appropriate for your individual circumstances and to monitor for any potential issues during treatment.

GLP-1 Receptor Agonists

Glucagon-like peptide-1 (GLP-1) receptor agonists are another class of medications that have shown promise in the management of CKD, particularly for patients with type 2 diabetes. These drugs mimic the effects of the hormone GLP-1, which stimulates insulin secretion, suppresses glucagon release, and slows gastric emptying. This results in better blood sugar control and additional benefits such as weight loss and reduced cardiovascular risk.

Recent studies have also demonstrated potential renal benefits of GLP-1 receptor agonists. The AWARD-7 trial published in The Lancet Diabetes & Endocrinology showed that dulaglutide, a GLP-1 receptor agonist, slowed the decline of kidney function in patients with type 2 diabetes and CKD compared to insulin glargine. Additionally, the trial found that dulaglutide reduced albuminuria, a key marker of kidney damage. (Source: https://www.thelancet.com/journals/landia/article/PIIS2213-8587(18)30060-5/fulltext)

GLP-1 Receptor Agonists include:
- Dulaglutide (Trulicity)
- Exenatide (Byetta, Bydureon)
- Liraglutide (Victoza, Saxenda)

- Lixisenatide (Adlyxin)
- Semaglutide (Ozempic, Rybelsus)

GLP-1 Receptor Agonists Drawbacks

Like all medications, GLP-1 receptor agonists can have drawbacks and potential side effects, which include:

Gastrointestinal side effects: GLP-1 receptor agonists can cause gastrointestinal issues such as nausea, vomiting, diarrhea, and constipation. These side effects are typically more common during the initial phase of treatment and may decrease over time.

Injection site reactions: Since GLP-1 receptor agonists are injectable medications, there's a possibility of experiencing pain, redness, or swelling at the injection site.

Hypoglycemia: While the risk of hypoglycemia (low blood sugar) is generally lower with GLP-1 receptor agonists compared to other diabetes medications, it can still occur, especially when used in combination with insulin or sulfonylureas.

Pancreatitis: Although rare, there have been reports of acute pancreatitis in people taking GLP-1 receptor agonists. Patients should be aware of the symptoms of pancreatitis and consult their healthcare provider if they suspect they might be experiencing it.

Allergic reactions: Some patients may experience allergic reactions to GLP-1 receptor agonists, which can include rash, itching, or difficulty breathing.

Cost and insurance coverage: GLP-1 receptor agonists can be expensive, and not all insurance plans may cover them. The cost and coverage can vary depending on the specific medication, the patient's insurance plan, and the availability of patient assistance programs or discounts.

Contraindications: GLP-1 receptor agonists are not recommended for people with a history of medullary thyroid carcinoma or multiple endocrine neoplasia syndrome type 2 due to a potential increased risk of thyroid cancer.

It's essential to discuss the potential risks and benefits of GLP-1 receptor agonists with your healthcare provider to determine if they are a suitable option for your specific situation. Your provider will help you weigh the potential drawbacks against the potential benefits for your kidney health and overall well-being.

Cost of GLP-1 Receptor Agonists

The affordability of GLP-1 (glucagon-like peptide-1) receptor agonists and their coverage by insurance can vary greatly depending on the specific medication, the patient's insurance plan, and the country in which the patient resides.

GLP-1 receptor agonists can be expensive, especially when compared to other diabetes medications. However, many insurance plans, including Medicare and Medicaid in the United States, do provide coverage for GLP-1 receptor agonists, but this can depend on the plan and the specific medication. It is essential to review your insurance plan to determine the extent of coverage and any potential out-of-pocket costs.

Some pharmaceutical companies offer patient assistance programs or discounts for those who cannot afford their medications or do not have insurance coverage. These programs can help eligible patients access GLP-1 receptor agonists at a reduced cost or even for free, depending on the specific program and eligibility criteria.

While GLP-1 receptor agonists can be expensive, many insurance plans do provide coverage for these medications. It is crucial to discuss the cost and insurance coverage with your healthcare provider and explore all available options to ensure you receive the most appropriate treatment for your specific situation.

HIF-PHD inhibitors (HIF-PHIs)

HIF-PHD inhibitors (HIF-PHIs) are a new class of medications designed to help people with chronic kidney disease (CKD). These drugs work by targeting a specific process in the body that responds to low oxygen levels, which is common in CKD patients.

In simpler terms, when oxygen levels are low, a protein called HIF helps the body adapt by promoting the production of red blood cells and improving blood flow. However, in people with CKD, this process is often disrupted. HIF-PHD inhibitors work by stabilizing the HIF protein, allowing the body to function better under low oxygen conditions.

For CKD patients, HIF-PHD inhibitors can help improve anemia, a common complication of kidney disease, by increasing the production of red blood cells. This can lead to better overall health and improved quality of life for those living with kidney disease. Jesduvroq (daprodustat) is one HIF-PHD inhibitor that has been approved in the U.S. to treat anemia in CKD patients.

The development of novel medications like SGLT-2 inhibitors, GLP-1 receptor agonists, and HIF-PHD inhibitors has opened up new avenues for CKD treatment. These drugs offer the potential to not only manage blood sugar in patients with diabetes and treat anemia but also to slow CKD progression and improve overall health. Best of all, these are only some of the advancements in kidney care – much more is on the way! As always, it is crucial for individuals with CKD to work closely with their healthcare team to determine the most appropriate treatment plan based on their unique needs and medical history.

EMOTIONAL AND MENTAL HEALTH SUPPORT

Living with chronic kidney disease (CKD) can be an emotional and mental challenge. The impact of the disease on daily life, uncertainty about its progression, and the need for ongoing medical care can lead to feelings of anxiety, depression, and stress. In this chapter, we will explore the importance of emotional and mental health support for individuals with CKD and their loved ones and provide strategies for coping with the emotional challenges that may arise during the course of the disease.

Understanding the Importance of Emotional and Mental Health Support

Maintaining good emotional and mental health is crucial for individuals with CKD, as it directly affects their ability to manage their condition and make important decisions about their treatment. Emotional well-being also plays a significant role in an individual's overall quality of life and ability to maintain relationships, engage in meaningful activities, and find joy and fulfillment in daily life.

Factors contributing to emotional and mental health challenges for individuals with CKD include:

- Physical symptoms and limitations associated with the disease

- The need for ongoing medical care and monitoring
- Uncertainty about the disease's progression and its impact on the future
- The potential need for dialysis or a kidney transplant
- The financial burden of medical expenses and potential loss of income
- The impact of the disease on relationships and social functioning

Given these challenges, it is essential for individuals with CKD and their loved ones to prioritize emotional and mental health support and develop coping strategies to help navigate the emotional landscape of living with a chronic illness.

Coping Strategies for Emotional Challenges

Acknowledge your feelings: It is natural to experience a range of emotions when living with CKD, such as fear, anger, sadness, frustration, and guilt. It is important to acknowledge these feelings and allow yourself to experience them without judgment. Recognizing your emotions can help you better understand your needs and seek appropriate support.

Seek professional help: If your emotions are overwhelming or interfering with your daily life, consider seeking support from a mental health professional, such as a psychologist or psychiatrist. They can provide counseling, therapy, and, if needed, medication to help manage anxiety, depression, or other mental health concerns.

Build a support network: Connecting with others who understand and empathize with your experience can be invaluable for maintaining emotional well-being. This support network can include friends, family, healthcare providers, and other individuals living with CKD. Support groups, both in-person and online, can provide a safe space to share your experiences, learn from others, and gain emotional support.

Practice self-care: Prioritizing your physical, emotional, and mental well-being is essential when living with CKD. Engage in activities that bring you joy and relaxation, such as hobbies, exercise, meditation, or spending time in nature. Maintain a healthy diet, get adequate sleep, and stay on top of your medical appointments and treatments.

Develop coping skills: Developing healthy coping strategies can help you manage the emotional challenges associated with CKD. Some effective coping strategies include deep breathing exercises, mindfulness meditation, progressive muscle relaxation, and journaling. Experiment with different strategies to find what works best for you.

Set realistic goals: Living with CKD may require adjustments to your lifestyle and expectations. Setting realistic goals can help you maintain a sense of purpose and control over your life while allowing for the flexibility needed to accommodate the demands of your condition.

Communicate with loved ones: Open communication with friends and family can help you express your needs, share your feelings, and gain emotional support. Be honest and clear about your experiences and challenges, as this can help your loved ones better understand your perspective and provide the support you need.

Educate yourself and others: Knowledge is empowering. Educate yourself about CKD, its progression, and treatment options to help alleviate some of the anxiety and uncertainty associated with the disease. Sharing this information with loved ones can also help them better understand your situation and provide appropriate support.

Seek financial assistance: The financial burden associated with CKD can be a significant source of stress for many individuals and families. Explore available resources and seek financial assistance, such as government programs, charitable organizations, or patient assistance programs, to help alleviate some of the financial strain.

Maintain a sense of humor: Laughter can be a powerful coping mechanism and an effective way to relieve stress. Finding humor in daily life, even in challenging situations, can help lighten the emotional load and provide a sense of perspective and resilience.

Supporting a Loved One with CKD

Family and friends play a vital role in the emotional well-being of individuals living with CKD. If you are a caregiver or loved one of someone with CKD, consider the following strategies to provide emotional and mental health support:

Be present and listen: Simply being there for your loved one, listening to their concerns and feelings, and offering empathy and understanding can be incredibly supportive. Avoid trying to "fix" their problems or dismiss their emotions; instead, validate their feelings and let them know you are there to support them.

Educate yourself: Learn about CKD and its impact on your loved one's life, so you can better understand their experiences and needs. This knowledge can help you provide more informed and empathetic support.

Encourage self-care and coping strategies: Encourage your loved one to prioritize their emotional well-being and engage in self-care activities and coping strategies that can help them manage stress and maintain a positive outlook.

Offer practical assistance: Offering help with daily tasks or medical appointments can alleviate some of the burden associated with CKD and allow your loved one to focus on their emotional well-being.

Be patient and flexible: Understand that living with CKD can be unpredictable and challenging, and be prepared to adapt to changes in your loved one's needs and circumstances. Practice patience and flexibility in your support.

Take care of yourself: As a caregiver or loved one, it is essential to prioritize your own emotional and mental health. Engage in self-care activities, seek support from friends or support groups, and consider counseling or therapy if needed. Remember that taking care of yourself enables you to provide better support for your loved one with CKD.

MANAGING CO-EXISTING CONDITIONS

Living with chronic kidney disease (CKD) is a challenging journey that requires continuous care and attention. In many cases, individuals with CKD may also have one or more co-existing conditions, which can further complicate their health management. In this chapter, we will explore some common co-existing conditions that individuals with CKD may encounter, and discuss strategies for managing these conditions in conjunction with CKD. This chapter will cover the following co-existing conditions:

- Diabetes
- Hypertension (high blood pressure)
- Cardiovascular disease
- Anemia
- Mineral and bone disorders
- Chronic lung diseases
- Depression and anxiety

Diabetes

Diabetes is a common co-existing condition among individuals with CKD. In fact, diabetes is the leading cause of CKD in many countries. When both diabetes and CKD are present, it is crucial to manage blood sugar levels carefully to prevent further kidney damage and complications related to diabetes.

Key strategies for managing diabetes in individuals with CKD include:

Monitoring blood sugar levels: Regularly monitoring blood sugar levels is crucial for individuals with both diabetes and CKD. This allows for timely adjustments in medications, diet, and lifestyle to maintain optimal blood sugar control.

Medication management: The choice of diabetes medications may need to be adjusted based on kidney function. Some diabetes medications may require dose adjustments or may be contraindicated in individuals with reduced kidney function. It is essential to consult with a healthcare provider to determine the most appropriate medication regimen for diabetes management in the context of CKD.

Diet modifications: A diet that is suitable for managing both diabetes and CKD should be followed. This diet may include controlling carbohydrate intake, choosing low-glycemic index foods, and monitoring protein, sodium, potassium, and phosphorus levels. A registered dietitian can provide personalized guidance for creating a meal plan that addresses the needs of both conditions.

Exercise: Regular physical activity can help improve blood sugar control, maintain a healthy weight, and reduce the risk of complications related to both diabetes and CKD. Consult with a healthcare provider to develop an appropriate exercise plan that takes into consideration any physical limitations or restrictions due to CKD.

Hypertension (High Blood Pressure)

Hypertension is another common co-existing condition in individuals with CKD. High blood pressure can cause further damage to the kidneys and increase the risk of cardiovascular complications. It is crucial to manage blood pressure effectively to slow the progression of CKD and reduce the risk of complications.

Key strategies for managing hypertension in individuals with CKD include:

Monitoring blood pressure: Regularly monitoring blood pressure at home can help individuals with CKD and hypertension stay informed about their condition and make necessary adjustments to medications, diet, and lifestyle.

Medication management: Several classes of blood pressure medications are available, and the choice of medication may depend on the severity of hypertension and the presence of other co-existing conditions. A healthcare provider will be able to recommend the most appropriate medication regimen for managing hypertension in the context of CKD.

Diet modifications: A diet that helps manage both CKD and hypertension should be followed. This diet may include reducing sodium intake, monitoring potassium and phosphorus levels, and maintaining a healthy weight. A registered dietitian can provide personalized guidance for creating a meal plan that addresses the needs of both conditions.

Exercise: Engaging in regular physical activity can help lower blood pressure, maintain a healthy weight, and improve overall cardiovascular health. Consult with a healthcare provider to develop an appropriate exercise plan that takes into consideration any physical limitations or restrictions due to CKD.

Cardiovascular Disease

Cardiovascular disease is a major complication and cause of death among individuals with CKD . The risk of cardiovascular disease increases as kidney function declines, making it essential to manage both CKD and cardiovascular risk factors simultaneously.

Key strategies for managing cardiovascular disease in individuals with CKD include:

Blood pressure control: As mentioned earlier, managing hypertension is crucial for individuals with CKD. Maintaining optimal blood pressure levels can help reduce the risk of cardiovascular events and slow the progression of CKD.

Cholesterol management: Elevated cholesterol levels can contribute to the development of cardiovascular disease. Monitoring cholesterol levels and implementing a heart-healthy diet and lifestyle changes can help manage cholesterol levels in individuals with CKD. In some cases, cholesterol-lowering medications, such as statins, may be prescribed by a healthcare provider.

Smoking cessation: Smoking is a significant risk factor for both cardiovascular disease and CKD progression. Quitting smoking can greatly reduce the risk of cardiovascular complications and improve overall health.

Weight management: Maintaining a healthy weight can help reduce the risk of cardiovascular disease and alleviate stress on the kidneys. A balanced diet and regular exercise, as recommended by a healthcare provider or dietitian, can help achieve and maintain a healthy weight.

Anemia

Anemia is a common complication of CKD, resulting from a reduction in the production of erythropoietin, a hormone that stimulates red blood cell production. Anemia can contribute to fatigue, weakness, and a decreased quality of life. For me, Anemia was the most challenging symptom to deal with, and I now keep a close eye on my hemoglobin (HB) lab results to prevent it from returning.

Key strategies for managing anemia in individuals with CKD include:

Monitoring hemoglobin levels: Regular monitoring of hemoglobin levels can help detect anemia early and initiate appropriate treatment.

Iron supplementation: Iron deficiency is a common cause of anemia in individuals with CKD. Oral or intravenous iron supplementation may be prescribed by a healthcare provider to address iron deficiency and improve anemia. TIP: Switch to cast iron cookware to boost the iron in your food.

Erythropoiesis-stimulating agents (ESAs): ESAs are medications that stimulate red blood cell production and may be prescribed to treat anemia in individuals with CKD. It is important to follow the healthcare provider's recommendations for the appropriate use and monitoring of ESAs.

Blood transfusions: In some cases, blood transfusions may be required to treat severe anemia in individuals with CKD. Healthcare providers will determine the necessity and timing of blood transfusions based on individual circumstances.

Mineral and Bone Disorders

Mineral and bone disorders (MBDs) are common complications of CKD, resulting from imbalances in calcium, phosphorus, and parathyroid hormone levels. MBDs can lead to bone pain, fractures, and vascular calcification.

Key strategies for managing MBDs in individuals with CKD include:

Monitoring mineral levels: Regular monitoring of calcium, phosphorus, and parathyroid hormone levels can help detect imbalances early and initiate appropriate treatment.

Phosphate binders: Phosphate binders are medications that help reduce the absorption of phosphorus from food, thus helping manage phosphorus levels in individuals with CKD. Healthcare providers will recommend the most appropriate type and dose of phosphate binders based on individual needs.

Vitamin D supplementation: Active vitamin D is essential for maintaining calcium and phosphorus balance in the body. Individuals with CKD may require vitamin D supplementation or active vitamin D analogs to help manage MBDs.

Dietary modifications: A diet that helps manage mineral and bone disorders should be followed. This diet may include controlling phosphorus intake, ensuring adequate calcium intake, and consuming foods rich in vitamin D. A registered dietitian can provide personalized guidance for creating a meal plan that addresses the needs of individuals with CKD and MBDs.

Chronic Lung Diseases

Chronic lung diseases, such as chronic obstructive pulmonary disease (COPD) and asthma, can co-exist with CKD and complicate overall health management. Proper management of chronic lung diseases is essential for maintaining the quality of life and preventing further complications.

Key strategies for managing chronic lung diseases in individuals with CKD include:

Monitoring lung function: Regular assessment of lung function through pulmonary function tests can help detect changes in lung disease progression and allow for timely adjustments in treatment.

Medication management: The choice of medications for chronic lung diseases may need to be adjusted based on kidney function. Some medications may require dose adjustments or may be contraindicated in individuals with reduced kidney function. It is essential to consult with a healthcare provider to determine the most appropriate medication regimen for managing chronic lung diseases in the context of CKD.

Stop Smoking: As mentioned earlier, smoking cessation is crucial for individuals with CKD and chronic lung diseases. Quitting smoking can significantly improve lung function and reduce the risk of complications related to both conditions.

Pulmonary rehabilitation: Pulmonary rehabilitation programs can help individuals with chronic lung diseases and CKD improve their exercise capacity, reduce symptoms, and enhance their quality of life. Consult with a healthcare provider to determine if pulmonary rehabilitation is appropriate and to develop a personalized plan.

Depression and Anxiety

As discussed in the previous chapter on emotional and psychological support, depression and anxiety are common co-existing conditions in individuals with CKD. These conditions can negatively impact overall health and well-being, making it essential to address and manage them effectively.

Key strategies for managing depression and anxiety in individuals with CKD include:

Professional help: Seeking support from mental health professionals, such as psychologists or psychiatrists, can provide valuable assistance in managing depression and anxiety. These professionals can offer counseling, therapy, and, if needed, medication to help address mental health concerns.

Support networks: Building and maintaining a support network of friends, family, healthcare providers, and fellow CKD patients can provide emotional support and understanding, helping to alleviate feelings of depression and anxiety.

Self-care: Prioritizing physical, emotional, and mental well-being is essential when living with CKD and depression or anxiety. Engaging in self-care activities, such as hobbies, exercise, meditation, or spending time in nature, can help improve overall emotional health.

Coping strategies: Developing healthy coping strategies, such as deep breathing exercises, mindfulness meditation, progressive muscle relaxation, and journaling, can help individuals with CKD and depression or anxiety manage their emotions more effectively.

THE IMPORTANCE OF BLOOD PRESSURE CONTROL

Blood pressure control is of utmost importance in managing chronic kidney disease (CKD). Uncontrolled blood pressure can exacerbate kidney damage, leading to a rapid decline in kidney function and increased risk of complications. As a kidney health coach, prioritizing blood pressure management is the first step in promoting better kidney health. This chapter will discuss the significance of blood pressure control in CKD, common medications used to manage blood pressure, and lifestyle changes that contribute to better blood pressure management.

The Impact of Blood Pressure Control on CKD

Hypertension, or high blood pressure, is both a cause and a consequence of CKD. Elevated blood pressure can damage blood vessels in the kidneys, impairing their ability to filter waste and regulate fluid balance effectively. This damage, in turn, contributes to a vicious cycle where impaired kidney function leads to further increases in blood pressure.

Proper blood pressure control is essential for the following reasons:

Slowing the progression of CKD: Controlling blood pressure can help reduce the rate at which kidney function declines, delaying the need for dialysis or a kidney transplant.

Reducing the risk of complications: Uncontrolled blood pressure increases the risk of cardiovascular events such as heart attacks, strokes, and heart failure. Managing blood pressure effectively can significantly reduce the risk of these life-threatening complications.

Preserving remaining kidney function: Blood pressure management helps protect the remaining healthy kidney tissue from further damage, maximizing the kidneys' ability to function despite the progression of CKD.

Improving the quality of life: Blood pressure control can help alleviate symptoms such as headaches, dizziness, and fatigue, leading to a better overall quality of life for individuals with CKD.

Blood Pressure Goals in CKD

The target blood pressure for individuals with CKD may vary depending on the specific circumstances and the presence of other co-existing conditions such as diabetes or cardiovascular disease. In general, a blood pressure target of less than 120/80 mmHg is recommended for most individuals with CKD. However, it is essential to consult with a healthcare provider to determine the most appropriate blood pressure goal for each individual.

Blood Pressure Medications in CKD

There are several classes of medications that can be used to manage blood pressure in individuals with CKD. These medications work through different mechanisms to lower blood pressure, and their choice may depend on factors such as kidney function, co-existing conditions, and potential side effects. The most commonly used blood pressure medications in CKD include:

Angiotensin-converting enzyme (ACE) inhibitors: These medications work by blocking the action of a hormone called angiotensin II, which narrows blood vessels and raises blood pressure. ACE inhibitors help relax blood vessels and lower blood pressure, thereby reducing the strain on the kidneys. Examples of ACE inhibitors include lisinopril, enalapril, and ramipril.

Angiotensin II receptor blockers (ARBs): ARBs also target the angiotensin II hormone but work by blocking its interaction with specific receptors on blood vessels. This action helps to dilate blood vessels, reduce blood pressure, and protect the kidneys. Examples of ARBs include losartan, valsartan, and irbesartan.

Calcium channel blockers: These medications work by preventing the entry of calcium into the cells of the heart and blood vessels, leading to relaxation of blood vessels and a reduction in blood pressure. Examples of calcium channel blockers include amlodipine, nifedipine, and diltiazem.

Diuretics: Also known as "water pills," diuretics help the kidneys eliminate excess sodium and water from the body, reducing blood volume and blood pressure. Examples of diuretics include hydrochlorothiazide, furosemide, and spironolactone.

Beta-blockers: These medications work by blocking the effects of adrenaline, a hormone that increases heart rate and blood pressure. By reducing the heart rate and the force of heart contractions, beta-blockers help lower blood pressure. Examples of beta-blockers include metoprolol, atenolol, and bisoprolol.

Alpha-blockers: Alpha-blockers work by relaxing the smooth muscle in blood vessels, leading to reduced blood pressure. Examples of alpha-blockers include doxazosin, prazosin, and terazosin.

It is important to note that many individuals with CKD may require a combination of medications to achieve optimal blood pressure control. A healthcare provider will determine the most appropriate medication regimen based on an individual's specific needs and circumstances.

Lifestyle Changes for Blood Pressure Control in

CKD

In addition to medications, adopting specific lifestyle changes can significantly contribute to blood pressure management in individuals with CKD. Some of the most impactful lifestyle modifications include:

Dietary changes: Adopting a kidney-friendly diet can help manage blood pressure by reducing sodium intake, promoting a healthy body weight, and improving overall cardiovascular health. The Dietary Approaches to Stop Hypertension (DASH) diet, which emphasizes whole grains, fruits, vegetables, lean proteins, and low-fat dairy products, has been shown to be particularly effective in lowering blood pressure.

Reducing sodium intake: Consuming excessive amounts of sodium can contribute to high blood pressure and fluid retention. Individuals with CKD should aim to limit their sodium intake to less than 2,300 mg per day or even lower, depending on the specific recommendations from their healthcare provider. Strategies for reducing sodium intake include cooking at home, using herbs and spices for flavoring instead of salt, and avoiding processed and fast foods high in sodium.

Regular physical activity: Engaging in regular physical activity can help lower blood pressure by promoting heart health, improving circulation, and reducing stress. Aim for at least 150 minutes of moderate-intensity aerobic exercise, such as brisk walking, swimming, or cycling, each week. Consult with a healthcare provider before starting a new exercise program to ensure that it is appropriate for your specific needs and limitations.

Weight management: Carrying excess weight, particularly around the abdomen, can contribute to high blood pressure. Losing even a small amount of weight can have a significant impact on blood pressure management. Consult with a healthcare provider or registered dietitian to develop a personalized weight loss plan that includes a balanced diet and regular physical activity.

Limiting alcohol consumption: Excessive alcohol intake can raise blood pressure and contribute to kidney damage. It is recommended that individuals with CKD limit their alcohol consumption to no more than one drink per day for women and two drinks per day for men.

Quitting Smoking: Smoking is a significant risk factor for high blood pressure and can worsen kidney damage. Quitting smoking can improve blood pressure control and overall kidney health.

Stress management: Chronic stress can contribute to elevated blood pressure. Developing healthy coping strategies, such as mindfulness meditation, deep breathing exercises, or engaging in hobbies, can help manage stress and improve overall well-being.

Regular monitoring: Regularly monitoring your blood pressure at home can help you and your healthcare provider track your progress and make adjustments to your treatment plan as needed. Keep a record of your blood pressure readings to share with your healthcare provider at your appointments.

When to Check Your Blood Pressure

Monitoring your blood pressure regularly is essential in managing chronic kidney disease and preventing complications. Here are some recommendations on when to check your blood pressure:

Routine monitoring: Check your blood pressure at least once a day, ideally at the same time each day. This helps establish a consistent routine and makes it easier to track trends or changes in your blood pressure over time.

Before taking blood pressure medications: It is crucial to check your blood pressure before taking any blood pressure medications, especially if you are feeling lightheaded or dizzy. If your blood pressure is low, consult your healthcare team before taking additional blood pressure medication. They may advise you to adjust your medication dosage or timing.

When experiencing symptoms: If you are feeling lightheaded, dizzy, or experiencing other symptoms that may be related to blood pressure fluctuations, it is important to check your blood pressure immediately. Keep a record of these readings and share them with your healthcare provider, as they can provide valuable insights into your blood pressure management.

After making lifestyle changes: If you have recently made significant lifestyle changes, such as starting a new exercise program, modifying your diet, or quitting smoking, it is helpful to monitor your blood pressure more frequently. This will help you understand the impact of these changes on your blood pressure and enable your healthcare team to make any necessary adjustments to your treatment plan.

At various times of the day: Occasionally, check your blood pressure at different times throughout the day. This can provide a more comprehensive picture of your blood pressure patterns and help identify any fluctuations related to daily activities, meals, or stress.

Remember, it is essential to use a properly calibrated and validated blood pressure monitor for accurate readings. Make sure to follow the manufacturer's instructions and your healthcare provider's recommendations on proper cuff size and positioning. Keep a log of your blood pressure readings, including the date, time, and any relevant notes, and share this information with your healthcare team during your appointments.

White Coat Syndrome: Understanding Its Impact on Blood Pressure

White Coat Syndrome, also known as White Coat Hypertension, is a phenomenon where a person's blood pressure is higher when measured in a medical setting, such as a doctor's office or hospital, compared to when measured at home or in other non-medical environments. This temporary increase in blood pressure is often attributed to anxiety or stress associated with visiting a healthcare provider.

Impact on Blood Pressure:

Anxiety-induced blood pressure elevation: The primary impact of White Coat Syndrome on blood pressure is the temporary increase caused by anxiety or stress related to the medical setting. This elevated blood pressure reading can make it difficult for healthcare providers to accurately assess a patient's blood pressure and determine the appropriate treatment.

Misdiagnosis or overtreatment: White Coat Syndrome can lead to a misdiagnosis of hypertension, as the elevated blood pressure readings in the medical setting may not accurately reflect a patient's true blood pressure levels. This can result in unnecessary treatment or medication for hypertension, which may cause side effects and additional healthcare costs.

Underestimating the severity of hypertension: Conversely, White Coat Syndrome can also result in underestimating the severity of a patient's hypertension, as their blood pressure may appear to be well-controlled in a medical setting but could be consistently elevated at home or in other environments.

Increased stress and anxiety: The fear of having high blood pressure readings in a medical setting can create a cycle of stress and anxiety for patients with White Coat Syndrome. This increased stress can further exacerbate blood pressure elevations, making it even more challenging to obtain accurate readings.

Managing White Coat Syndrome:

To minimize the impact of White Coat Syndrome on blood pressure management, consider the following strategies:

Home blood pressure monitoring: Regularly monitoring your

blood pressure at home can provide a more accurate picture of your true blood pressure levels, as it captures readings in a familiar and comfortable environment. Share these readings with your healthcare provider to help them better understand your blood pressure patterns and make more informed treatment decisions.

Relaxation techniques: Practicing relaxation techniques, such as deep breathing exercises or mindfulness meditation, can help reduce anxiety and stress associated with medical visits. Incorporate these techniques before and during your appointments to help minimize the impact of White Coat Syndrome on your blood pressure readings.

Develop a trusting relationship with your healthcare provider: Establishing a strong rapport and open communication with your healthcare provider can help alleviate anxiety related to medical visits. Discuss your concerns about White Coat Syndrome with them, and work together to develop strategies for managing this phenomenon.

Ambulatory blood pressure monitoring: In some cases, your healthcare provider may recommend ambulatory blood pressure monitoring, which involves wearing a small blood pressure device that continuously records your blood pressure over a 24-hour period. This method can provide a more comprehensive understanding of your blood pressure patterns and help determine whether you have true hypertension or White Coat Syndrome.

By understanding White Coat Syndrome and its impact on blood pressure, you can work with your healthcare provider to develop strategies to minimize its effects and ensure accurate blood pressure management.

CREATININE AND YOUR KIDNEYS

Creatinine: What's the Big Deal?

So, you've probably heard about creatinine and how it's connected to kidney health. But what's the real story? Creatinine is a waste product that comes from the regular breakdown of muscle tissue in our bodies. While it's true that creatinine levels can give us a rough idea of how well our kidneys are filtering waste, it's essential to understand that creatinine itself isn't the bad guy. It's merely an indicator, and focusing solely on reducing creatinine won't necessarily improve kidney function.

The Creatinine-Kidney Connection: Debunking the Myth

A lot of kidney patients might think that if they just lower their creatinine levels, they'll magically improve their kidney function. However, that's not quite how it works. Creatinine is just a marker, not the root cause of kidney problems. Let's use a wild example to make this point crystal clear: imagine someone amputating their legs. Sure, their creatinine levels would likely drop because of the decreased muscle mass, but does that mean their kidneys are suddenly functioning better? Absolutely not.

Kidney Health: The Real Deal

Now that we've cleared up the creatinine confusion, let's talk about what kidney patients should really focus on: living a heart-healthy lifestyle and making diet and lifestyle changes as recommended by their healthcare team. This approach is way more effective in slowing down the progression of kidney disease. Here's what that looks like:

Diet: Hook up with a renal dietitian who can help you create a tasty, kidney-friendly meal plan that fits your unique dietary needs. Look for foods that pack a nutritional punch without loading you down with sodium, potassium, or phosphorus.

Exercise: Don't forget to get moving! Regular physical activity, as advised by your healthcare team, can help you maintain a healthy weight, keep your blood pressure in check, and boost your overall wellbeing.

Blood pressure management: Speaking of blood pressure, make sure you're keeping an eye on it. Work with your healthcare team to develop a plan that keeps your blood pressure in the healthy zone through medication, diet, and lifestyle changes.

Medication adherence: Stick to your healthcare team's recommendations when it comes to medications. Take them as directed and let your team know if you're experiencing any side effects.

Stress reduction: Chill out with some stress reduction techniques, like meditation, deep breathing exercises, or enjoying hobbies that bring you joy. After all, chronic stress can wreak havoc on your overall health, including your kidneys.

In a nutshell, it's time to stop worrying about creatinine as the enemy. It's just a marker, and focusing on it alone won't improve kidney health. Instead, prioritize living a heart-healthy lifestyle and making the right diet and lifestyle changes to keep your kidneys in tip-top shape.

IS KIDNEY FAILURE IN YOUR FUTURE

It's natural to feel concerned about the possibility of kidney failure after being diagnosed with Chronic Kidney Disease (CKD). However, it's essential to understand that only a small percentage of people with CKD will ultimately require dialysis. By taking appropriate steps, many patients can manage their kidney health and slow down the progression of their CKD.

CKD Stage 3: According to a study published in the Journal of the American Society of Nephrology, around 1.3% of patients with CKD Stage 3 progressed to kidney failure requiring dialysis or transplantation within five years. (Source: https://jasn.asnjournals.org/content/21/6/1058)

To better understand your risk of kidney failure, we recommend using the Kidney Failure Risk website (**https://kidneyfailurerisk.com**). This helpful tool can provide an estimate of your personal risk of progressing to kidney failure, which requires dialysis or kidney transplantation. As you read through this chapter, we aim to ease your concerns by shedding light on the factors that influence CKD progression and empowering you with knowledge and practical strategies to maintain your kidney health. Remember, knowledge is power, and staying informed can help you take control of your CKD journey.

Predicting Future CKD Risks

While there is no guaranteed method for predicting future CKD risks, the following chart can give you an idea of the risk level based on your eGFR and protein in the urine, or you can access an interactive kidney failure risk factor tool at https://kidneyfailurerisk.com/

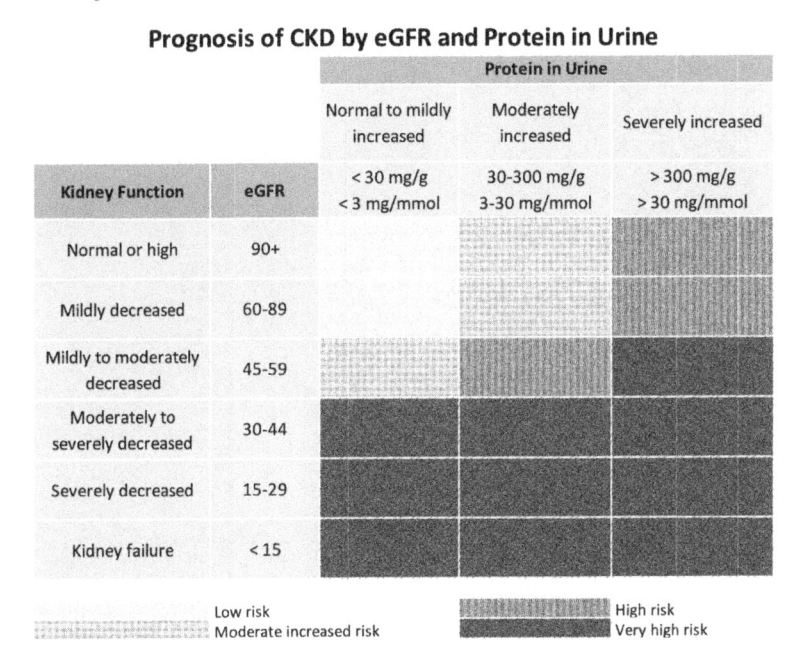

Prognosis of CKD by eGFR and Protein in Urine

Kidney Function	eGFR	Protein in Urine: Normal to mildly increased (< 30 mg/g, < 3 mg/mmol)	Moderately increased (30-300 mg/g, 3-30 mg/mmol)	Severely increased (> 300 mg/g, > 30 mg/mmol)
Normal or high	90+	Low risk	Moderate increased risk	High risk
Mildly decreased	60-89	Low risk	Moderate increased risk	High risk
Mildly to moderately decreased	45-59	Moderate increased risk	High risk	Very high risk
Moderately to severely decreased	30-44	High risk	Very high risk	Very high risk
Severely decreased	15-29	Very high risk	Very high risk	Very high risk
Kidney failure	< 15	Very high risk	Very high risk	Very high risk

Low risk
Moderate increased risk
High risk
Very high risk

Monitoring eGFR and Protein Leakage in CKD Management

Regular monitoring of eGFR and protein leakage is essential in managing CKD. Assessing these factors can help healthcare providers:

1. Track the progression of CKD
2. Evaluate the effectiveness of treatments aimed at preserving kidney function
3. Detect complications associated with CKD, such as cardiovascular disease

4. Make timely adjustments to treatment plans

DIALYSIS

Dialysis is a medical treatment that replicates some of the functions of the kidneys when they are no longer able to perform them adequately. It is primarily used for individuals with chronic kidney disease (CKD), particularly those in the advanced stages, and also for patients with acute kidney injury (AKI) who require temporary assistance while their kidneys recover.

What is Dialysis

Dialysis is a life-sustaining therapy that helps to filter waste products, excess fluids, and electrolytes from the bloodstream when the kidneys cannot perform these tasks effectively. There are two main types of dialysis: hemodialysis and peritoneal dialysis. Both types aim to maintain the balance of chemicals and fluids within the body, helping patients with kidney dysfunction maintain their health.

When is Dialysis Used

Dialysis is often recommended for patients with end-stage renal disease (ESRD) when their kidney function has declined to the point where it can no longer sustain life. This typically occurs when the eGFR falls below 5-7. Dialysis can also be used for patients with acute kidney injury (AKI), where sudden damage to the kidneys results in a temporary loss of function. In such cases, dialysis serves as a supportive measure, allowing the kidneys time to recover.

How Does Dialysis Work

Hemodialysis: Hemodialysis is the most common type of

dialysis. It involves the use of a dialysis machine and an artificial kidney, called a dialyzer, to filter the patient's blood. During treatment, the blood is circulated through the dialyzer, where a semi-permeable membrane separates the blood from a dialysate solution. Waste products, excess fluids, and electrolytes pass through the membrane and into the dialysate solution, while the cleaned blood is returned to the patient's body. Hemodialysis treatments are typically performed three times per week and last for about 3-4 hours per session.

Peritoneal Dialysis: Peritoneal dialysis uses the patient's own peritoneum, the lining of the abdomen, as a natural filter. A catheter is surgically implanted into the abdomen, allowing dialysate solution to be introduced into the peritoneal cavity. Waste products and excess fluids pass through the peritoneal membrane and into the dialysate solution, which is then drained from the body. Peritoneal dialysis can be performed as continuous ambulatory peritoneal dialysis (CAPD), where exchanges are done manually several times a day, or as automated peritoneal dialysis (APD), where a machine performs the exchanges overnight.

Both types of dialysis help to alleviate the symptoms and complications associated with kidney dysfunction. The choice between hemodialysis and peritoneal dialysis depends on various factors, such as the patient's overall health, lifestyle, and personal preferences. It is essential to discuss these options with your healthcare team to determine the best treatment approach for your situation.

Determining the Right Time for Dialysis

The decision to start dialysis is often based on several factors, including kidney function, symptoms, nutritional status, co-existing conditions, and patient preferences.

Kidney Function: Kidney function is typically measured by the estimated glomerular filtration rate (eGFR). Healthcare providers generally recommend initiating dialysis when the eGFR falls below 5-7 or when the individual begins to experience significant symptoms related to kidney failure. Research shows that starting dialysis early does not improve outcomes or life expectancy.

Symptoms and Quality of Life: Symptoms such as fatigue, nausea, swelling, difficulty breathing, and cognitive impairment may indicate the need for dialysis. The impact of these symptoms on an individual's quality of life is a significant factor in the decision to start dialysis.

Nutritional Status: Malnutrition is common in individuals with advanced CKD and can contribute to poor outcomes. If an individual cannot maintain adequate nutrition due to their kidney disease, healthcare providers may recommend starting dialysis.

Co-existing Conditions: The presence of other medical conditions, such as heart disease, diabetes, or high blood pressure, can influence the decision to start dialysis. In some cases, initiating dialysis may help manage these co-existing conditions and improve overall health.

Patient Preferences: The decision to start dialysis should be made collaboratively between the individual, their healthcare providers, and their support system. Personal preferences, lifestyle factors, and treatment goals are essential considerations in this decision-making process.

The Dialysis Process: Preparation and Monitoring

Before starting dialysis, patients undergo a thorough evaluation by their healthcare team, including nephrologists, nurses, and dietitians. They will discuss the different types of dialysis, the required preparations, and potential complications, to help the patient make an informed decision about their treatment plan.

Once dialysis is initiated, ongoing monitoring and regular lab tests are crucial to ensure optimal treatment outcomes.

These tests help the healthcare team assess the patient's overall health, track the effectiveness of the dialysis, and make any necessary adjustments to the treatment plan. This may include changes in dialysis frequency, duration, or the dialysate solution composition.

Dialysis and Lifestyle Adjustments

While dialysis can greatly improve the quality of life for patients with advanced kidney disease, it requires significant lifestyle adjustments. Adhering to a strict diet and fluid restrictions is essential to maintaining proper electrolyte balance and minimizing complications. Patients must also consider the time commitment involved in dialysis treatments and make arrangements for transportation to and from dialysis centers if they opt for hemodialysis.

For those who choose peritoneal dialysis, there will be a learning curve in managing their treatment independently or with the assistance of a caregiver. In either case, it is crucial to maintain good hygiene and cleanliness during the dialysis process to minimize the risk of infection.

Dialysis as a Bridge to Transplantation

Dialysis is not a cure for kidney disease, but it can help maintain a patient's health until they receive a kidney transplant, which is often the best long-term treatment option. Transplantation can offer a better quality of life, as it allows patients to regain many of their normal activities and reduce dietary restrictions. However, the availability of donor kidneys is limited, and patients must meet certain eligibility criteria to be considered for transplantation. While waiting for a transplant, patients should maintain open communication with their healthcare team to optimize their dialysis treatment and overall health.

KIDNEY TRANSPLANT

A kidney transplant is a life-changing surgical procedure in which a healthy kidney from a living or deceased donor is placed into the body of a person with end-stage renal disease (ESRD). This new kidney takes over the functions of the person's failed kidneys, allowing them to lead a healthier life free from the need for dialysis. In this chapter, we will discuss various aspects of kidney transplantation, including eligibility criteria, the process itself, and post-transplant considerations.

Kidneys for transplantation come from two main sources: living donors and deceased donors. Living donors are usually close family members or friends who have a compatible blood type and tissue match. Deceased donors are individuals who have recently passed away and had agreed to donate their organs for transplantation. In both cases, the donated kidney undergoes rigorous testing to ensure its suitability for transplantation.

To be eligible for a kidney transplant, a person must have ESRD, be in good overall health, and be able to adhere to a strict post-transplant medication regimen. Age is not a strict factor, as kidney transplants have been performed on patients ranging from infants to older adults. However, the patient's overall health and the potential risks and benefits are taken into consideration.

In some cases, a person may undergo more than one kidney transplant in their lifetime if the first transplant fails or if the transplanted kidney loses its function after several years. However, multiple transplants may be limited by the availability of suitable donors and the patient's overall health.

Certain factors may disqualify a person from receiving a kidney transplant, such as active infections, cancer, severe heart or lung disease, or a history of noncompliance with medical treatment. The transplant team will evaluate each patient's specific circumstances to determine their eligibility.

During a kidney transplant, the surgeon places the new kidney in the lower abdomen, connecting it to the recipient's blood vessels and bladder. The patient's own failed kidneys are usually left in place unless they pose a risk due to infection or other complications.

It is essential to remember that a kidney transplant is not a cure for kidney disease, but rather a treatment option that can improve the patient's quality of life. After the transplant, the patient will need to take immunosuppressive medications to prevent their immune system from attacking the new kidney. Regular follow-up appointments with their healthcare team will also be necessary to monitor their progress and overall health.

Benefits and Risks of Kidney Transplantation

Benefits: A successful kidney transplant can significantly enhance an individual's quality of life by alleviating many symptoms associated with CKD, such as fatigue, nausea, and difficulty concentrating. Transplant recipients often experience fewer dietary restrictions and enjoy greater flexibility in their daily routines compared to those on dialysis. Furthermore, kidney transplantation is linked to a lower risk of cardiovascular disease and longer life expectancy than remaining on dialysis.

Risks: Kidney transplantation carries several risks, including transplant rejection, infections, and complications resulting from the surgery itself. Transplant recipients must take immunosuppressive medications to prevent rejection, which can lead to side effects and increase the risk of infections and certain cancers. It is crucial for individuals considering a kidney transplant to discuss the potential benefits and risks with their healthcare providers.

The Transplant Evaluation Process

Referral: The transplant process begins with a referral from a nephrologist or dialysis care team to a transplant center, which typically occurs when an individual's kidney function declines to a point where a transplant may soon become necessary.

Medical evaluation: The transplant center will conduct a thorough medical evaluation to determine if an individual is a suitable candidate for a kidney transplant. This evaluation includes a comprehensive assessment of the individual's overall health, kidney function, and any co-existing medical conditions that could impact the transplant's success or pose additional risks.

Psychosocial evaluation: A psychosocial evaluation assesses an individual's mental health, social support system, and ability to adhere to the complex medical regimen required after transplantation. This evaluation may involve interviews with a social worker, psychologist, or psychiatrist.

Financial evaluation: A financial evaluation helps ensure that the individual has the necessary resources to cover the costs associated with transplantation and post-transplant care, including medications, follow-up appointments, and potential travel expenses.

Transplant listing: If an individual is deemed an appropriate candidate for a kidney transplant, they will be placed on a waiting list for a deceased donor organ. The waiting time for a kidney transplant can vary widely, depending on factors such as blood type, tissue type, and geographic location.

Living Donor Transplantation

Advantages: Living donor kidney transplantation offers several advantages over deceased donor transplantation, including shorter waiting times, better organ quality, and improved long-term graft survival. Additionally, living donor transplants can be scheduled, allowing for better preparation and coordination between the donor and recipient.

Eligibility: Living donors must be in good overall health and have normal kidney function. A comprehensive medical evaluation is performed to assess the potential donor's health and ensure that the donation will not pose undue risks to the donor or recipient.

Types of living donor transplantation: There are several types of living donor transplantation, including directed donation (where the donor specifies the intended recipient) and non-directed donation (where the donor does not specify a recipient and the organ is allocated through the usual transplant waiting list). Paired kidney exchange programs are also available, in which two or more donor-recipient pairs who are not compatible with each other can swap donors to enable compatible transplants.

Post-Transplant Care

Immunosuppressive medications: Transplant recipients must take immunosuppressive medications for the life of the transplanted kidney to prevent rejection. These medications can have side effects and may require adjustments over time to maintain the appropriate balance between preventing rejection and minimizing risks associated with immunosuppression.

Monitoring and follow-up: Regular follow-up appointments with the transplant team are crucial for monitoring kidney function, detecting potential complications, and ensuring the success of the transplant. Blood tests, imaging studies, and biopsies of the transplanted kidney may be required at various intervals to assess graft function and detect signs of rejection or infection.

Lifestyle modifications: Maintaining a healthy lifestyle is

essential for transplant recipients. This includes adhering to a balanced diet, engaging in regular physical activity, and avoiding tobacco, excessive alcohol consumption, and illicit drug use. Transplant recipients should also take precautions to minimize their risk of infections, such as practicing good hygiene, avoiding large crowds during periods of high infection risk, and staying up-to-date on vaccinations.

Managing co-existing conditions: It is important for transplant recipients to continue managing any co-existing medical conditions, such as diabetes or high blood pressure, which can impact the health of the transplanted kidney and overall well-being. Regular appointments with healthcare providers and adherence to prescribed medications are essential for managing these conditions.

Emotional and mental health support: The transplant process can be emotionally challenging, and some individuals may experience feelings of anxiety, depression, or guilt. Support from healthcare providers, mental health professionals, support groups, and loved ones can help transplant recipients navigate these emotions and maintain a positive outlook on their health and well-being.

Transplant Rejection

Types of rejection: There are three main types of transplant rejection: hyperacute rejection, which occurs within minutes to hours of the transplant; acute rejection, which typically occurs within days to weeks following the transplant; and chronic rejection, which develops over months to years after the transplant. Rejection can be caused by various factors, including the recipient's immune system attacking the transplanted kidney, inadequate immunosuppression, or non-adherence to medications.

Signs and symptoms: Signs of transplant rejection may include a sudden decrease in urine output, swelling in the legs or ankles, unexplained weight gain, fever, pain or tenderness at the transplant site, or elevated blood pressure. It is important for transplant recipients to be vigilant for these signs and symptoms and report any concerns to their healthcare providers promptly.

Treatment: Treatment for transplant rejection depends on the type and severity of the rejection. In some cases, adjusting immunosuppressive medications or administering additional medications to suppress the immune system may be sufficient to manage the rejection. In more severe cases, treatments such as plasmapheresis or intravenous immunoglobulin may be required. In some instances, if the rejection cannot be reversed, the transplanted kidney may fail, necessitating a return to dialysis and potential consideration for another transplant.

A kidney transplant can offer many benefits for individuals with chronic kidney disease, including improved quality of life and increased life expectancy. It is essential to weigh the potential benefits and risks, undergo a thorough evaluation process, and consider living donor transplantation options. Post-transplant care, including lifestyle modifications and managing co-existing conditions, is vital for ensuring the long-term success of the transplant.

TIPS FOR FINDING AN ORGAN DONOR

Finding an organ donor, particularly for a kidney transplant, can be a challenging and emotionally taxing journey. However, there are several strategies and resources available to help increase your chances of finding a suitable living donor. This chapter will provide tips for spreading the word in your community and introduce you to the Living Kidney Donors Network's free service, "Having Your Kidney Donor Find You," which can aid in your search for a living kidney donor.

1. Share Your Story

One of the most effective ways to find a potential organ donor is by sharing your story with those around you. By opening up about your need for a transplant, you can raise awareness and inspire others to consider becoming a living donor.

- Talk to family and friends: Your loved ones can be your strongest advocates. Share your journey with them and ask for their support in spreading the word.
- Use social media: Platforms such as Facebook, Twitter, and Instagram can be powerful tools for reaching a wider audience. Create posts that detail your story, and encourage your network to share them with their own connections.
- Write a letter or email: Consider sending a heartfelt

letter or email to your extended network, including colleagues, acquaintances, and members of social or religious organizations you are part of.

2. Engage Your Community

Involving your local community can help amplify your message and increase the likelihood of finding a donor.

- Organize community events: Plan events such as fundraisers, awareness walks, or educational seminars to draw attention to your cause and educate the public about living organ donation.
- Contact local media: Reach out to newspapers, radio stations, and TV channels to share your story and request coverage or interviews.
- Partner with local organizations: Collaborate with community groups, schools, and religious institutions to raise awareness and create a support network.

3. Create a Website or Blog

Creating a personal website or blog can be an effective way to document your journey, provide updates, and share information about living organ donation.

- Choose a platform: There are several user-friendly website builders, such as TheGreatSocialExperiment.net, Wix, Weebly, or WordPress, that can help you create a professional-looking site without coding knowledge.
- Share your story: Write blog posts detailing your experiences, progress, and any challenges you face. This can help humanize your story and create a connection with potential donors.
- Provide resources: Include information about the organ donation process, the benefits of living

donation, and how someone can become a living donor for you.

4. Utilize Online Support Networks

Online support networks can connect you with others who have faced similar challenges and provide additional resources for finding an organ donor.

- Join support groups: Participate in online forums or social media groups dedicated to organ transplantation and living organ donation.
- Leverage existing networks: Reach out to organizations such as the National Kidney Foundation, American Transplant Foundation, or Donate Life America for guidance and resources.

5. Having Your Kidney Donor Find You

The Living Kidney Donors Network's free service, "Having Your Kidney Donor Find You" (https://havingyourkidneydonorfindyou.org/), is a valuable resource designed to help individuals in need of a kidney transplant connect with potential living donors.

- Register for the service: Complete a simple online registration form to get started.
- Create a personal profile: Develop a profile that includes your story, photos, and any relevant medical information.
- Share your profile: Use the unique link provided by the service to share your profile with your network and encourage others to do the same.

6. Attend Workshops and Seminars

Many organizations and transplant centers offer workshops and seminars designed to educate individuals about living organ donation and provide tools for finding a donor.

- Research local workshops: Check the websites of nearby transplant centers, hospitals, or nonprofit organizations to see if they offer any workshops or seminars.

- Attend events: Participate in these educational events and use the opportunity to network with others in similar situations and professionals who can offer guidance.

- Apply learned strategies: Implement the tips and strategies you learn at these events to enhance your search for a living donor.

7. Consider Paired Kidney Exchanges

If you have a willing but incompatible donor, consider participating in a paired kidney exchange program. These programs facilitate the exchange of donors between incompatible donor-recipient pairs, increasing the chances of finding a compatible donor.

- Research paired exchange programs: Look for well-established paired exchange programs, such as the National Kidney Registry (https://www.kidneyregistry.org/), Alliance for Paired Kidney Donation, or United Network for Organ Sharing (UNOS) Kidney Paired Donation Pilot Program.

- Register with a program: After discussing with your transplant team, register with a suitable paired exchange program to increase your chances of finding a compatible donor.

8. Maintain Open Communication with Your Healthcare Team

Your healthcare providers can be valuable allies in your search for a living organ donor. They possess a wealth of knowledge and experience that can be invaluable in guiding you through the process.

- Keep them informed: Regularly update your healthcare team about your efforts to find a donor and seek their input or advice.
- Ask for referrals: Inquire if your healthcare team can recommend any resources, events, or organizations that could aid in your search for a donor.

Finding a living organ donor can be a complex and emotional journey. By utilizing the tips and resources outlined in this chapter, you can greatly improve your chances of finding a suitable donor and moving forward with a life-changing transplant. Always remember to stay patient, persistent, and positive throughout the process, and lean on the support of your loved ones and healthcare team.

CONSERVATIVE MANAGEMENT OF KIDNEY FAILURE

End-stage renal disease (ESRD), also known as kidney failure, is a critical condition where the kidneys are no longer able to perform their essential functions. Dialysis and kidney transplantation have been the traditional treatment options for ESRD. However, conservative management has emerged as a viable alternative for some patients, particularly those who may not be suitable candidates for dialysis or transplantation due to factors such as age, comorbidities, or personal preferences.

Conservative management is a comprehensive approach to treating kidney failure that focuses on symptom control, preserving kidney function, and enhancing the quality of life. In this chapter, we will delve into the components of conservative management, the benefits and drawbacks of this approach, and the factors to consider when determining if conservative management is the right choice for you or a loved one.

Components of Conservative Management

Medical Management: Medical management within conservative care is a personalized and holistic approach, tailored to the individual needs of the patient. It may include the use of medications to control blood pressure, blood sugar levels, and electrolyte imbalances. Additional medications may be prescribed to manage kidney-related complications such as anemia, bone mineral disorders, and acidosis. Regular monitoring of kidney function and overall health through laboratory tests and clinical assessments is also a crucial aspect of medical management.

Nutritional Management: A well-balanced diet is an essential component of conservative management. Collaborating with a renal dietitian allows patients to develop a personalized meal plan that addresses their unique nutritional needs while considering factors such as taste preferences, cultural practices, and lifestyle. Nutritional management may involve monitoring and adjusting the intake of protein, sodium, potassium, phosphorus, and fluids to help preserve kidney function, control symptoms, and prevent complications.

Symptom Management: Kidney failure can result in a wide range of symptoms, such as fatigue, nausea, itching, and difficulty sleeping. Symptom management in conservative care focuses on alleviating these symptoms through a combination of medical treatments, lifestyle modifications, and complementary therapies. Techniques such as relaxation exercises, meditation, or acupuncture may be employed to manage symptoms and improve overall well-being.

Psychosocial Support: Living with kidney failure can take a significant toll on an individual's mental and emotional well-being. Conservative management emphasizes the importance of providing comprehensive psychosocial support to patients and their families. This may include individual or group counseling, support groups, and assistance with navigating the healthcare system and coordinating care. Encouraging open communication and fostering strong support networks can help patients cope with the challenges of kidney failure and enhance their quality of life.

Advance Care Planning: Advance care planning is a critical aspect of conservative management, as it allows patients to express their preferences for their future care and make informed decisions about their treatment options. Patients should engage in ongoing conversations with their healthcare team and loved ones to ensure that their wishes are understood and respected, and that appropriate plans are in place to address their medical, emotional, and practical needs.

Benefits and Drawbacks of Conservative Management

Benefits:

Improved Quality of Life: Conservative management aims to enhance the quality of life for patients by addressing their physical, emotional, and social needs. Many patients who opt for conservative management report a greater sense of control over their care and a higher overall satisfaction with their treatment experience.

Avoidance of Dialysis or Transplantation: For some patients, dialysis or transplantation may not be the preferred treatment option due to various factors such as age, comorbidities, or personal preferences. Conservative management offers an alternative approach that focuses on preserving kidney function and managing symptoms without the need for dialysis or transplantation.

Cost-Effectiveness: Conservative management can be a more cost-effective approach to treating kidney failure, as it typically involves fewer hospitalizations, invasive procedures, and long-term medical expenses associated with dialysis or transplantation. Additionally, conservative management can help patients avoid the financial burden and stress related to the ongoing costs of dialysis treatment or post-transplant care.

Drawbacks:

Potential for Disease Progression: While conservative management focuses on preserving kidney function, it may not prevent the progression of kidney disease in some cases. As kidney function declines, patients may experience more severe symptoms and complications that can negatively impact their quality of life.

Limited Treatment Options: Conservative management may not be suitable for all patients, particularly those with rapidly progressing kidney disease or severe complications. In such cases, dialysis or transplantation may be the only viable treatment options to manage the disease effectively.

Need for Continuous Monitoring and Adjustments: Conservative management requires ongoing monitoring of kidney function and overall health, as well as regular adjustments to medications, diet, and lifestyle factors. This can be time-consuming and may place a significant burden on patients and their families.

Determining if Conservative Management is Right for You

Deciding whether conservative management is an appropriate treatment option for you or a loved one requires careful consideration of various factors, including the stage of kidney disease, overall health, personal preferences, and quality of life goals. It is essential to engage in open and honest discussions with your healthcare team about your treatment options, potential benefits and drawbacks, and long-term expectations.

When considering conservative management, it may be helpful to:

Consult with a multidisciplinary team of healthcare professionals, including nephrologists, renal dietitians, social workers, and psychologists, to gain a comprehensive understanding of your condition and the available treatment options.

Discuss your personal goals, values, and preferences with your healthcare team to ensure that your chosen treatment approach aligns with your unique needs and desires.

Seek the input and support of family members, friends, or support groups, as they can provide valuable insights and encouragement during the decision-making process.

Stay informed about the latest research and advancements in kidney disease management to ensure that you are making the most informed decisions about your care.

Continuously reevaluate your treatment plan and make adjustments as needed, in collaboration with your healthcare team, to ensure that your chosen approach remains effective and appropriate for your changing needs and circumstances.

Conservative management is a comprehensive and holistic approach to treating kidney failure that focuses on symptom control, preserving kidney function, and enhancing the quality of life. By carefully considering the benefits and drawbacks of conservative management, as well as consulting with a multidisciplinary team of healthcare professionals, patients can make informed decisions about their treatment options and work towards achieving the best possible outcomes for their unique circumstances.

DIET AND NUTRITION FOR KIDNEY HEALTH

Maintaining a healthy diet is essential for individuals with kidney disease, as it can help slow down the progression of the disease, manage symptoms, and improve overall health. Kidney patients often feel a loss of control over their treatment, but diet is one area where they can regain control and actively participate in their healthcare. However, navigating the complexities of diet and nutrition can be overwhelming for many kidney patients, leading to confusion and uncertainty about what to eat. In this chapter, we will discuss the role of a renal dietitian and why working with one can empower kidney patients to feel confident in their food choices.

The Role of a Renal Dietitian

A renal dietitian is a healthcare professional who specializes in the nutritional management of kidney disease. They have the expertise and training to provide personalized dietary recommendations tailored to an individual's specific needs, taking into account their kidney function, other medical conditions, and overall health goals. Some of the key roles and responsibilities of a renal dietitian include:

Assessment: A renal dietitian will assess a patient's nutritional status, medical history, and dietary habits to develop a comprehensive understanding of their unique needs and challenges. This assessment may involve reviewing laboratory results, discussing symptoms and medications, and evaluating the patient's current diet.

Education: A crucial aspect of a renal dietitian's role is educating patients about the relationship between diet and kidney health. They will provide information on the importance of various nutrients, such as protein, potassium, phosphorus, and sodium, and how they affect kidney function. The dietitian will also explain the potential risks and benefits of different dietary choices, empowering patients to make informed decisions about their food intake.

Personalized dietary planning: Based on the assessment and education, a renal dietitian will work with the patient to develop a personalized meal plan that meets their nutritional needs, preferences, and lifestyle. This meal plan will take into consideration any dietary restrictions or modifications necessary to manage kidney disease and its associated symptoms.

Monitoring and adjusting: A renal dietitian will regularly monitor a patient's progress, laboratory results, and overall health to determine if any adjustments to their dietary plan are needed. They will work closely with the patient and their healthcare team to make any necessary changes and ensure optimal nutritional management.

Support and motivation: Living with kidney disease and adhering to a specialized diet can be challenging, both emotionally and practically. A renal dietitian provides ongoing support, encouragement, and guidance to help patients overcome these challenges and maintain a healthy, kidney-friendly diet.

Why Work with a Renal Dietitian?

Working with a renal dietitian offers several benefits for kidney patients, including:

Expertise in kidney health: Renal dietitians have specialized knowledge and training in the field of kidney health, making them uniquely qualified to provide dietary recommendations tailored to the specific needs of kidney patients.

Personalized approach: Each individual with kidney disease has unique nutritional needs and challenges. A renal dietitian will work closely with the patient to develop a personalized meal plan that meets their specific requirements, preferences, and lifestyle.

Confidence in food choices: By providing education and guidance on the relationship between diet and kidney health, a renal dietitian can help patients feel more confident and knowledgeable about their food choices, enabling them to take control of their health.

Better management of kidney disease: A renal dietitian can help patients manage their kidney disease more effectively by providing dietary strategies to slow down the progression of the disease, manage symptoms, and improve overall health.

Coordination with the healthcare team: A renal dietitian works closely with the patient's healthcare team to ensure that the dietary plan aligns with the overall treatment plan and to address any potential interactions between medications and food.

Nutrient Considerations for Kidney Health

When working with a renal dietitian, kidney patients will learn about various nutrients that play a role in kidney health. Some of these nutrients **may** need to be restricted or monitored, depending on the individual's kidney function and overall health. It is important to note that any food restrictions should come from the patient's healthcare team, as nutrients like potassium are protective of the heart and kidneys and should only be restricted when they can no longer be managed by the kidneys. Some of the key nutrients to consider include:

Protein: Protein is an essential nutrient for the body's growth, repair, and maintenance. However, in some cases, kidney patients may need to limit their protein intake to reduce the workload on the kidneys and prevent further kidney damage. A renal dietitian can help determine the appropriate amount of protein for each patient and suggest high-quality protein sources.

Potassium: Potassium is a mineral that plays a vital role in maintaining proper nerve and muscle function. While it is protective of the heart and kidneys, in individuals with advanced kidney disease, the kidneys may not be able to remove excess potassium from the blood, leading to high potassium levels (hyperkalemia). A renal dietitian can provide guidance on the appropriate potassium intake and help patients choose potassium-rich foods that can be safely included in their diet.

Phosphorus: Phosphorus is another essential mineral that helps maintain healthy bones and teeth, among other functions. However, in individuals with kidney disease, the kidneys may not effectively remove excess phosphorus from the blood, leading to high phosphorus levels (hyperphosphatemia). A renal dietitian can help patients manage their phosphorus intake by suggesting phosphorus-rich foods to avoid and recommending phosphorus binders, if needed.

Sodium: Sodium is an essential mineral that helps regulate fluid balance and blood pressure. However, excessive sodium intake can lead to high blood pressure and further damage the kidneys. A renal dietitian can help patients manage their sodium intake by suggesting low-sodium alternatives, providing tips for reading food labels, and offering strategies for reducing sodium intake when dining out.

Fluids: In some cases, kidney patients **may** need to monitor their fluid intake to prevent fluid overload, which can lead to swelling, high blood pressure, and strain on the heart. A renal dietitian can help patients determine the appropriate amount of fluid intake and provide guidance on how to manage fluid consumption throughout the day.

Lifestyle Changes to Support Kidney Health

In addition to working with a renal dietitian, kidney patients can also make several lifestyle changes to support their kidney health. Some of these changes include:

Maintain a healthy weight: Achieving and maintaining a healthy weight can help reduce the risk of high blood pressure, diabetes, and other conditions that can lead to kidney damage.

Exercise regularly: Engaging in regular physical activity can help improve cardiovascular health, maintain a healthy weight, and manage stress, all of which can benefit kidney health.

Quit smoking: Smoking can cause damage to blood vessels and decrease blood flow to the kidneys, leading to a decline in kidney function. Quitting smoking can significantly improve kidney and overall health.

Limit alcohol consumption: Excessive alcohol consumption can contribute to high blood pressure and kidney damage. It is recommended to limit alcohol intake to moderate levels.

Manage stress: Chronic stress can negatively affect blood pressure and overall health, including kidney function. Practicing stress management techniques, such as deep breathing exercises, meditation, or yoga, can help promote kidney health.

Diet and nutrition play a crucial role in kidney health, and working with a renal dietitian can empower kidney patients to take control of their health through informed food choices. By understanding the importance of various nutrients, seeking guidance from a renal dietitian, and adopting a personalized approach to meal planning, patients can feel confident in their ability to manage their kidney disease and maintain their overall well-being. In addition to dietary changes, incorporating healthy lifestyle habits, such as maintaining a healthy weight, exercising regularly, quitting smoking, limiting alcohol consumption, and managing stress, can further support kidney health and improve the patient's quality of life. By actively participating in their healthcare and taking control of their diet, kidney patients can make a significant difference in the management and progression of their kidney disease.

PHOSPHORUS

Phosphorus is an essential mineral found in many foods and plays a crucial role in maintaining overall health. It is important for bone health, muscle function, nerve function, and the production of energy in the body. However, in individuals with kidney disease, managing phosphorus levels becomes critical, as impaired kidney function can lead to an imbalance in phosphorus levels, which may cause further complications. In this chapter, we will discuss the importance of understanding phosphorus in the context of kidney disease, the differences between natural and added phosphorus, and how to identify phosphorus additives on food labels.

The Importance of Phosphorus Management in Kidney Disease

Healthy kidneys play a vital role in regulating the balance of phosphorus in the body. However, when kidney function declines due to kidney disease, the kidneys may become less efficient at removing excess phosphorus from the blood. As a result, phosphorus levels can become too high, a condition known as hyperphosphatemia.

Elevated phosphorus levels can cause several health issues, including:

Weakening of bones: High phosphorus levels can lead to a decrease in calcium levels, as the body tries to maintain a proper balance between these two minerals. This imbalance can result in the weakening of bones and an increased risk of fractures.

Calcification of tissues: Excess phosphorus can cause calcium to build up in blood vessels, heart valves, and other tissues, leading to calcification. This can impair the function of these tissues and increase the risk of cardiovascular events.

Hormonal imbalance: High phosphorus levels can disrupt the balance of hormones responsible for regulating calcium and phosphorus levels in the body, such as parathyroid hormone (PTH). This can lead to secondary hyperparathyroidism, which can exacerbate bone loss and increase the risk of cardiovascular complications.

Given these potential health risks, it is crucial for individuals with kidney disease to manage their phosphorus intake and maintain appropriate phosphorus levels in the body.

Natural vs. Added Phosphorus

Phosphorus can be found in two forms in our diet: natural phosphorus and added phosphorus.

Natural phosphorus: This is the phosphorus naturally present in various food sources, such as meat, poultry, fish, dairy products, beans, nuts, and whole grains. Our body absorbs approximately 40-60% of the natural phosphorus present in these foods. Since the absorption rate is not very high, it is generally safe for individuals with kidney disease to consume foods containing natural phosphorus, as long as they are mindful of portion sizes and follow the guidance of their healthcare team.

Added phosphorus: This is the phosphorus added to processed and packaged foods in the form of phosphorus-containing additives. These additives are often used as preservatives, stabilizers, or emulsifiers to improve the texture, shelf life, and flavor of food products. The absorption rate of added phosphorus is much higher than natural phosphorus, with the body absorbing up to 90% of it. As a result, consuming foods with added phosphorus can significantly contribute to elevated phosphorus levels in individuals with kidney disease, and it is essential to limit the intake of such foods.

Identifying Phosphorus Additives on Food Labels

To manage phosphorus intake effectively, it is essential to read food labels and identify products containing phosphorus additives. Here are some tips to help you spot these additives:

1. Look for words containing "PHOS": When reading the ingredients list on food labels, look for words containing the letters "PHOS." This is a common indicator that a phosphorus-containing additive is present in the product. Some examples of phosphorus additives include:

    - Sodium phosphate
    - Calcium phosphate
    - Potassium phosphate
    - Dicalcium phosphate
    - Tricalcium phosphate
    - Tetrasodium pyrophosphate
    - Disodium phosphate
    - Monosodium phosphate

2. Be cautious with processed and packaged foods: Phosphorus additives are commonly found in processed and packaged foods such as canned soups, processed meats, frozen meals, baked goods, and snack foods. It is essential to read the ingredient list of these products carefully and opt for alternatives with lower phosphorus content or no added phosphorus whenever possible.

3. Opt for fresh and unprocessed foods: Fresh fruits, vegetables, and minimally processed grains are generally low in phosphorus and free of phosphorus additives. Incorporating more of these foods into your diet can help you manage your phosphorus

intake and promote overall kidney health.

4. Limit the consumption of fast food and restaurant meals: Many fast food and restaurant meals contain high amounts of added phosphorus, as well as other nutrients that can be harmful to kidney health, such as sodium and potassium. Limiting the consumption of these meals and choosing home-cooked options can help you better control your phosphorus intake.

5. Consult a renal dietitian: A renal dietitian can provide personalized guidance on managing phosphorus intake based on your specific needs and kidney function. They can help you understand food labels, identify phosphorus additives, and create a balanced meal plan that supports your kidney health.

Common High Phosphorus Foods and Drinks

Dairy products: Milk, cheese, yogurt, and other dairy products are significant sources of phosphorus. Some dairy alternatives, such as almond or soy milk, may also have added phosphates.

Meat and poultry: Beef, chicken, turkey, and pork contain naturally occurring phosphorus. Processed meats, such as deli meats, sausages, and hot dogs, can have even higher levels due to added phosphates.

Fish and seafood: Fish like salmon, tuna, and halibut, as well as shellfish like shrimp and scallops, are high in phosphorus.

Nuts and seeds: Almonds, peanuts, sunflower seeds, and pumpkin seeds are high in phosphorus. Nut butters, such as peanut butter and almond butter, also contain significant amounts of phosphorus.

Beans and legumes: Kidney beans, lentils, chickpeas, and other legumes are rich in phosphorus.

Whole grains: Whole grain products like whole wheat bread, brown rice, and whole grain pasta contain more phosphorus than their refined counterparts.

Carbonated beverages: Dark-colored sodas and other carbonated beverages often contain phosphoric acid, a phosphorus-containing additive.

Processed foods: Many processed and packaged foods, such as frozen meals, canned soups, and snack foods, contain phosphorus additives. It is essential to read the ingredient list of these products carefully and opt for alternatives with lower phosphorus content or no added phosphorus whenever possible.

Phosphorus Binders

Phosphorus binders are medications that help control the level of phosphorus in the blood, particularly for people with kidney disease. When the kidneys are not functioning properly, they may not be able to effectively remove excess phosphorus from the body. High phosphorus levels can lead to various health issues, such as bone disorders, calcification of tissues, and an increased risk of cardiovascular disease.

Phosphorus binders work by binding to phosphorus in the gastrointestinal tract, preventing its absorption into the bloodstream. Instead, the phosphorus is eliminated from the body through the digestive system in the form of feces. This helps to maintain a healthy phosphorus balance in the body.

There are several types of phosphorus binders available, including:

Calcium-based binders: These binders, such as calcium carbonate (Tums) and calcium acetate (Phoslo), contain calcium that binds to phosphorus in the gut. While effective, they can sometimes lead to an excess intake of calcium, which could cause hypercalcemia or increased risk of vascular calcification.

Non-calcium-based binders: These binders do not contain calcium and are less likely to cause issues related to high calcium levels. Examples include sevelamer (Renvela, Renagel) and lanthanum carbonate (Fosrenol). Sevelamer is a polymer that binds phosphorus without adding calcium, while lanthanum carbonate is a metal-based compound that also effectively binds phosphorus.

Iron-based binders: These medications, such as sucroferric oxyhydroxide (Velphoro) and ferric citrate (Auryxia), contain iron that binds to phosphorus. Iron-based binders have the added benefit of helping to manage iron levels in people with kidney disease, who often suffer from anemia.

It's important to note that phosphorus binders should be taken under the guidance of a healthcare professional, as individual needs may vary. These medications are often taken with meals, as this is when phosphorus intake typically occurs. Your healthcare provider will determine the appropriate type and dosage of phosphorus binder based on your kidney function, phosphorus levels, and other individual factors.

Managing phosphorus intake is an essential aspect of maintaining kidney health for individuals with kidney disease. By understanding the differences between natural and added phosphorus, learning how to identify phosphorus additives on food labels, and working with a renal dietitian, you can take control of your diet and make informed choices that support your kidney health. Remember, always consult your healthcare team before making any significant changes to your diet, as they can provide personalized guidance based on your unique medical needs and circumstances.

POTASSIUM

Potassium is an essential mineral and electrolyte that plays a crucial role in maintaining proper muscle, nerve, and heart function. However, when kidney function declines, the ability to filter and maintain a proper balance of potassium may be compromised. In this chapter, we will discuss the importance of potassium in kidney disease and provide tips for managing potassium intake, emphasizing that potassium should only be restricted if your healthcare team or dietitian instructs you to do so.

The role of potassium in kidney health

Potassium is necessary for many bodily functions, including:

- Regulating fluid balance
- Supporting proper nerve and muscle function, including the heart
- Maintaining healthy blood pressure

For individuals with healthy kidney function, excess potassium is filtered out and excreted through urine. However, when kidney function is impaired, the kidneys may not be able to remove potassium effectively, leading to a buildup of potassium in the blood. This condition is known as hyperkalemia, which can be dangerous and cause irregular heart rhythms or even heart failure.

On the other hand, potassium has been shown to have protective effects on both the heart and kidneys when managed properly. For those with kidney disease, it's important not to restrict potassium unnecessarily and to work closely with your healthcare team or dietitian to ensure you're consuming the right amount of potassium for your needs.

Tips for managing potassium intake

Consult with your healthcare team or dietitian: Before making any changes to your potassium intake, consult with your healthcare team or dietitian. They will assess your kidney function, blood potassium levels, and other factors to determine the appropriate amount of potassium for your needs.

Understand food sources of potassium: Educate yourself on foods that are high and low in potassium. High-potassium foods include bananas, oranges, tomatoes, potatoes, spinach, and avocados. Lower-potassium options include apples, grapes, berries, green beans, and zucchini. Familiarize yourself with the potassium content of various foods so you can make informed choices.

Monitor portion sizes: If you need to limit potassium, be mindful of portion sizes for high-potassium foods. Eating smaller amounts of these foods can help you manage your potassium intake without completely eliminating them from your diet.

Leach high-potassium vegetables: Leaching is a process that can help reduce the potassium content of certain high-potassium vegetables, like potatoes. To leach, cut vegetables into small pieces, soak them in a large amount of water for at least two hours (or overnight), and then drain and rinse before cooking.

Choose lower-potassium fruits and vegetables: Incorporate more low-potassium fruits and vegetables into your diet to help manage potassium intake. These foods can still provide essential nutrients and fiber without contributing excessively to your potassium levels.

Limit high-potassium beverages: Some beverages, such as fruit juices and sports drinks, can be high in potassium. Opt for water, herbal tea, or other lower-potassium options to stay hydrated without increasing potassium levels.

Read food labels: Some processed foods may contain added potassium, often in the form of potassium chloride. Read food labels carefully to avoid consuming excessive amounts of potassium from these sources.

Regularly monitor blood potassium levels: Work closely with your healthcare team to monitor your blood potassium levels regularly. This will help ensure you're maintaining a healthy balance and can adjust your diet as needed.

Medications to reduce potassium

Sodium polystyrene sulfonate (Kayexalate): This medication helps lower high potassium levels by binding with potassium in the gut, allowing it to be eliminated through the digestive system. It is typically taken orally or used as an enema.

Patiromer (Veltassa): This oral medication also works by binding potassium in the gut and promoting its excretion. It is often used for the long-term treatment of hyperkalemia in patients with chronic kidney disease.

Sodium zirconium cyclosilicate (Lokelma): Similar to the other potassium binders, sodium zirconium cyclosilicate works by trapping potassium in the gut and promoting its elimination. It is also taken orally.

Loop diuretics (e.g., furosemide, bumetanide, torsemide): These medications help the kidneys excrete more potassium in the urine by increasing the amount of water and sodium that is filtered out of the blood.

Blood pressure medications that can increase potassium

Angiotensin-converting enzyme (ACE) inhibitors (e.g., lisinopril, enalapril, ramipril): These medications help lower blood pressure by blocking the production of angiotensin II, a hormone that narrows blood vessels and increases blood pressure. However, ACE inhibitors can also cause the kidneys to retain more potassium, potentially leading to higher potassium levels in the blood.

Angiotensin II receptor blockers (ARBs) (e.g., losartan, valsartan, candesartan): Like ACE inhibitors, ARBs lower blood pressure by blocking the effects of angiotensin II on blood vessels. They can also cause the kidneys to retain more potassium.

Potassium-sparing diuretics (e.g., spironolactone, eplerenone, amiloride, triamterene): Unlike loop diuretics, potassium-sparing diuretics help the kidneys excrete more water and sodium while preserving potassium levels. They are used to treat high blood pressure and heart failure but can lead to higher potassium levels in the blood.

Potassium plays an essential role in maintaining overall health, particularly for those with kidney disease. It's important not to restrict potassium unnecessarily, as it can have protective effects on both the heart and kidneys when managed properly. Always consult with your healthcare team or dietitian before making changes to your potassium intake and follow their guidance on managing potassium levels tailored to your individual needs.

Remember, maintaining a well-balanced diet is crucial for overall health and kidney function. By understanding the potassium content of various foods, monitoring portion sizes, and working closely with your healthcare team or dietitian, you can take control of your potassium intake and make informed decisions about your diet.

SODIUM

Managing sodium intake is a critical aspect of kidney health, especially for those with kidney disease. As a kidney health coach, I always emphasize the importance of sodium management when planning meals. Sodium intake directly affects blood pressure control, which is crucial for kidney patients. In this chapter, we'll explore the relationship between sodium and kidney disease, providing guidance on how to manage sodium intake effectively.

Sodium and Its Role in the Body

Sodium is an essential mineral primarily found in the blood and extracellular fluid in the body. It helps regulate fluid balance by attracting water to areas with high sodium concentration. This process helps maintain proper blood volume and blood pressure, which is essential for the proper functioning of the heart and kidneys. Sodium is also crucial for nerve impulse transmission and muscle contraction.

Kidney Disease and Sodium

In healthy individuals, the kidneys effectively filter excess sodium from the bloodstream and excrete it through urine. However, when kidney function is impaired due to chronic kidney disease (CKD), the kidneys may not be able to eliminate excess sodium as efficiently. This can lead to sodium retention, causing fluid buildup and increased blood pressure. High blood pressure, also known as hypertension, is both a cause and a complication of kidney disease. Uncontrolled hypertension can further damage the kidneys and accelerate the progression of

CKD.

Excess sodium intake can also contribute to other health issues commonly associated with kidney disease, such as heart disease, stroke, and edema (swelling due to fluid retention).

Sodium Intake Recommendations for Kidney Disease

The American Heart Association (AHA) recommends that most adults should consume no more than 2,300 milligrams (mg) of sodium per day, with an ideal limit of 1,500 mg per day for those with high blood pressure or other risk factors for heart disease. For individuals with kidney disease, sodium intake recommendations may vary depending on the stage of the disease, overall health, and other factors. Your healthcare team will provide personalized guidance on the appropriate sodium intake for your specific situation.

Strategies for Managing Sodium Intake

Read food labels: Processed and packaged foods are often high in sodium. Read food labels to check the sodium content of products and choose lower-sodium alternatives when possible.

Choose fresh, whole foods: Opt for fresh fruits, vegetables, and unprocessed meats, as they are generally lower in sodium than their processed counterparts.

Cook at home: Preparing meals at home allows you to control the amount of sodium in your dishes. Use fresh ingredients and limit the use of high-sodium condiments, sauces, and seasonings.

Limit processed foods: Processed foods, such as canned soups, frozen meals, and snack foods, are often high in sodium. Limit your consumption of these foods and opt for lower-sodium alternatives when possible.

Be cautious when dining out: Restaurant meals can be high in sodium. Request that your meal be prepared without added salt, and choose dishes with lower-sodium ingredients, such as grilled or steamed vegetables, lean proteins, and whole grains.

Use herbs and spices for flavor: Enhance the flavor of your meals with herbs, spices, and other low-sodium seasonings, such as garlic, onion, lemon juice, and vinegar.

Rinse canned foods: Rinsing canned vegetables, beans, and other foods can help reduce their sodium content.

Practice portion control: Consuming smaller portions of high-sodium foods can help limit your overall sodium intake.

Monitor your fluid intake: Consuming an appropriate amount of fluids can help prevent fluid retention and maintain proper blood pressure. Consult your healthcare team for personalized recommendations on daily fluid intake.

Educate yourself and others: Share information about sodium and kidney disease with family and friends, as they can play an essential role in supporting your dietary changes and maintaining a low-sodium environment.

Track your sodium intake: Keep a food diary to track your daily sodium intake. This can help you identify sources of excess sodium in your diet and make necessary adjustments.

Gradually reduce sodium: If you're used to consuming a high-sodium diet, it may take time for your taste buds to adjust to lower-sodium foods. Gradually reduce your sodium intake to help your body adapt to the change.

Consult with a dietitian: A registered dietitian specializing in kidney disease can help you develop a personalized meal plan that meets your nutritional needs while managing sodium intake effectively.

Monitor your blood pressure: Regularly monitoring your blood pressure can help you identify potential issues related to sodium intake and kidney disease. Work with your healthcare team to establish a blood pressure monitoring routine and set appropriate targets.

Be proactive about your kidney health: In addition to managing sodium intake, focus on other aspects of kidney health, such as maintaining a healthy weight, managing blood sugar levels, staying active, and adhering to your prescribed medications.

Salt Alternatives and Hidden Potassium

For kidney patients trying to reduce their sodium intake, it's common to seek salt alternatives to enhance the flavor of their food. However, it's important to be aware that some salt substitutes may contain potassium, which can be a concern for those on a potassium-restricted diet. In this section, we will discuss some common salt alternatives and their potential impact on potassium levels.

Potassium-based salt substitutes: Many salt substitutes on the market are potassium-based, using potassium chloride as the primary ingredient. These products can be a significant source of potassium, which may not be suitable for kidney patients with a potassium restriction. It is essential to read the ingredient labels carefully before using any salt substitute and consult with your healthcare team or dietitian before incorporating them into your diet.

Herbs and spices: Natural herbs and spices are an excellent way to add flavor to your meals without adding sodium or potassium. Examples include garlic, onion, basil, oregano, rosemary, thyme, and parsley. Additionally, incorporating citrus juices, such as lemon or lime juice, and vinegar can enhance the taste without negatively impacting potassium levels.

Blends without potassium: Some salt-free seasoning blends do not contain potassium and can be used as a safe alternative for those on a potassium-restricted diet. Brands like Dash (formerly Mrs. Dash) offer a variety of sodium-free and potassium-free seasoning blends that can help add flavor to your meals without increasing your potassium intake. Always check the label to ensure that the blend you choose does not contain potassium.

Be cautious with "lite" salts: "Lite" salts or low-sodium salts are a mixture of sodium chloride and potassium chloride. While they contain less sodium than regular table salt, they still provide potassium, which may not be appropriate for those on a potassium-restricted diet. As with other salt substitutes, read the ingredient labels carefully and consult with your healthcare team or dietitian before using these products.

Challenges in Managing Sodium Intake

Despite the importance of managing sodium intake for individuals with kidney disease, several challenges may arise. Some individuals may find it difficult to adjust to a low-sodium diet due to taste preferences or the ubiquity of high-sodium foods in the modern diet. Additionally, the hidden sodium content in many processed foods can make it challenging to accurately track sodium intake. Overcoming these challenges may require ongoing support from healthcare professionals, family members, and peers, as well as a commitment to making lasting dietary changes.

PROTEIN AND CKD

Protein is an essential nutrient that plays a vital role in maintaining and repairing the body's cells and tissues. For those with Chronic Kidney Disease (CKD), understanding the importance of protein and how to manage its intake is crucial.

In this chapter, we will delve into what protein is, its significance for the body, and its particular relevance for CKD patients. Furthermore, we will discuss the different types of protein, including animal and plant-based sources.

What is Protein

Protein is a macronutrient made up of smaller units called amino acids, which are the building blocks of our body. It plays a critical role in numerous bodily functions, including growth, repair, and maintenance of muscles, bones, skin, and other tissues. Protein also serves as a component of enzymes, hormones, and antibodies, ensuring proper functioning and regulation of various processes within the body.

The Importance of Protein for CKD Patients

For individuals with CKD, it's essential to strike a balance in protein intake. Consuming an appropriate amount of protein can help preserve muscle mass and support overall health, while avoiding excessive intake that can strain the kidneys further.

As kidney function declines, the body's ability to process protein waste products is diminished, causing these waste products to accumulate in the bloodstream. A carefully planned diet that manages protein consumption can help alleviate this burden on the kidneys and potentially slow down the progression of CKD.

Types of Protein: Animal and Plant Sources

There are two primary types of protein sources: animal-based and plant-based. Animal-based proteins, found in meat, poultry, fish, dairy products, and eggs, are considered complete proteins because they provide all the essential amino acids that the body cannot produce on its own.

On the other hand, plant-based proteins come from sources such as legumes, nuts, seeds, and whole grains. While many plant-based proteins are considered incomplete, as they may lack one or more essential amino acids, combining various plant-based protein sources can still provide all the necessary amino acids for optimal health.

For CKD patients, incorporating more plant-based protein sources may have additional benefits, as these proteins tend to be less taxing on the kidneys compared to animal-based proteins. Additionally, plant-based diets often have higher fiber content and lower levels of saturated fats, which can contribute to improved cardiovascular health and overall well-being.

Why Plant Sources Are Better

Plant-based proteins are considered to be less taxing on the kidneys for several reasons:

Lower Acid Load: Plant-based proteins typically have a lower acid load compared to animal-based proteins. The metabolic breakdown of animal proteins produces a higher amount of acid in the body, which the kidneys must filter and remove. Over time, a consistently high acid load can contribute to a condition called metabolic acidosis and cause further stress on the kidneys. In contrast, plant-based proteins tend to produce fewer acidic by-products, resulting in a reduced burden on the kidneys.

Lower Phosphorus Content: Animal-based proteins are

known to have a higher phosphorus content, which can be problematic for individuals with CKD. When the kidneys are not functioning efficiently, they struggle to remove excess phosphorus from the blood, leading to an elevated phosphorus level. High blood phosphorus can contribute to bone and heart problems. Plant-based proteins, on the other hand, generally contain lower amounts of phosphorus. Moreover, the phosphorus found in plant-based proteins is less bioavailable, meaning that the body absorbs it less efficiently, further reducing the phosphorus burden on the kidneys.

Reduced Proteinuria: Studies have shown that a plant-based diet can help lower proteinuria, which is the presence of excess protein in the urine. Proteinuria is a common symptom of kidney disease, and reducing it can help protect the kidneys from further damage. Plant-based proteins are less likely to contribute to proteinuria, as they are more easily metabolized and filtered by the kidneys compared to animal proteins.

Improved Blood Pressure and Cardiovascular Health: Plant-based diets have been linked to lower blood pressure and improved cardiovascular health, both of which are essential for CKD patients. High blood pressure can exacerbate kidney damage, while cardiovascular diseases are a common complication in people with kidney disease. Consuming more plant-based proteins, along with whole grains, fruits, vegetables, and legumes, can help support a heart-healthy lifestyle and reduce stress on the kidneys.

Reduced Hyperfiltration: Consuming animal-based proteins has been linked to a phenomenon called hyperfiltration, which occurs when the kidneys are forced to work harder than usual to filter and remove waste products from the bloodstream. This increased workload can put additional stress on the kidneys and accelerate the progression of kidney disease. Plant-based proteins are less likely to cause hyperfiltration, as they tend to be more easily metabolized and filtered by the kidneys. This results in less strain on the kidneys and helps protect them from

further damage.
Determining the Right Amount of Protein

When it comes to protein intake, it's essential to understand that there is no one-size-fits-all approach. The appropriate amount of protein for an individual with CKD depends on various factors, such as their age, weight, activity level, overall health, and the stage of their kidney disease.

To determine the right amount of protein for your specific needs, it's crucial to consult with your health care team or a renal dietitian. They will assess your unique circumstances and help you establish an individualized protein intake plan tailored to your requirements. Your dietitian may also monitor and adjust your protein consumption based on your lab results and the progression of your kidney disease.

Remember, it's important to maintain a balanced diet and work closely with your health care team to ensure you're getting the necessary nutrients while also protecting your kidneys. Trusting the guidance of professionals will empower you to make informed choices about your protein intake and overall dietary plan.

FIBER

In the world of kidney health, fiber doesn't often make it into the limelight. But as the unsung hero of nutrition, it's time to give fiber the recognition it deserves, and maybe share a chuckle or two along the way!

The Role of Fiber in Kidney Disease

Fiber is a type of carbohydrate that your body can't digest, which means it passes through your digestive system without being broken down. This may not sound glamorous, but it does some pretty fabulous things for your body. For people with kidney disease, fiber can help improve bowel function, reduce inflammation, lower blood pressure, and even help maintain better blood sugar levels.

The Benefits of Fiber

When it comes to kidney health, fiber has a few tricks up its sleeve. Research has shown that a higher fiber intake is associated with improved kidney function and a slower progression of kidney disease. One study published in the American Journal of Kidney Diseases found that people with CKD who consumed a higher-fiber diet had a 30% lower risk of developing end-stage renal disease (ESRD) and a 27% lower risk of death compared to those with lower fiber intakes (1). Fiber can also help to lower cholesterol levels, reducing the risk of heart disease, which is a common complication for those with kidney disease.

"Fiber-rific" Food Sources

Now that you're on board the fiber train, let's talk about

where to find it. The best sources of fiber are whole plant-based foods, like fruits, vegetables, whole grains, nuts, and seeds. Some kidney-friendly high-fiber options include:

- Apples and pears (with skin)
- Berries
- Green beans and peas
- Leafy greens
- Whole-grain bread, pasta, and cereals
- Brown rice and quinoa
- Nuts and seeds (in moderation due to their high phosphorus content)

Remember, not all fruits and veggies are created equal when it comes to kidney health, so be sure to consult your renal dietitian for personalized recommendations.

Fiber Supplements: Friend or Foe?

Sometimes, getting enough fiber through food alone can be a challenge. This is where fiber supplements come in handy. There are many types of fiber supplements available, including psyllium husk, inulin, and methylcellulose. While these supplements can be beneficial, it's essential to start slow and gradually increase your intake to prevent gastrointestinal discomfort (and any embarrassing moments!). Be sure to talk to your healthcare team before adding any supplements to your diet, as some may interact with medications or affect your nutrient levels.

How Much Fiber Is Enough

The recommended daily intake of fiber varies depending on age and gender. According to the Institute of Medicine, the following daily fiber recommendations apply:

- Men aged 19-50 years: 38 grams

- Men aged 51 years and older: 30 grams
- Women aged 19-50 years: 25 grams
- Women aged 51 years and older: 21 grams

However, it's essential to keep in mind that these recommendations are for the general population, and individuals with kidney disease should consult their healthcare team or renal dietitian for personalized advice on fiber intake.

Tips to Increase Fiber without Gassing Up

When it comes to increasing fiber intake, it's crucial to do so gradually to avoid gastrointestinal discomfort, such as bloating, gas, and diarrhea. Here are some steps to help you increase your fiber intake safely and effectively:

1. Start slow: Begin by adding a small amount of fiber-rich foods to your meals. This could be as simple as adding a side of steamed vegetables or a small fruit salad to your lunch or dinner.

2. Gradual increase: Over the course of a few weeks, gradually increase the amount of fiber in your diet by incorporating more high-fiber foods into your meals and snacks.

3. Drink plenty of water: As you increase your fiber intake, it's essential to drink plenty of water to help the fiber move through your digestive system and prevent constipation.

4. Pay attention to your body: Monitor how your body reacts to the increased fiber intake. If you experience gastrointestinal discomfort, consider slowing down the pace at which you're adding fiber to your diet.

5. Consult your healthcare team: If you have kidney disease or other medical conditions, it's essential to consult with your healthcare team or renal dietitian

before making significant changes to your diet, including increasing your fiber intake.

By following these steps, you can safely increase your fiber intake and enjoy the numerous health benefits associated with a fiber-rich diet while minimizing any potential side effects.

Laughing Our Way to Better Health

Fiber might be a bit of a shy topic, but there's no reason we can't have a little fun with it. After all, it's doing us a world of good! So, the next time you find yourself in a conversation about kidney health, don't forget to give fiber a shout-out. And remember, a little bit of humor can go a long way in breaking down barriers and helping us embrace the benefits of fiber for a healthier, happier life with kidney disease.

References:

Kelly, J. T., Palmer, S. C., Wai, S. N., Ruospo, M., Carrero, J. J., Campbell, K. L., & Strippoli, G. F. (2016). Healthy Dietary Patterns and Risk of Mortality and ESRD in CKD: A Meta-Analysis of Cohort Studies. American Journal of Kidney Diseases, 69(2), 260-268.

GUT HEALTH

Gut health plays a crucial role in maintaining overall health, and this is especially true for individuals living with chronic kidney disease (CKD). A healthy gut can positively influence your immune system, metabolism, and nutrient absorption, all of which can impact your kidney function. In this chapter, we will discuss the significance of gut health in CKD, explore the benefits of probiotics and prebiotics, and provide recommendations for incorporating gut-friendly foods into your diet.

The Connection Between Gut Health and Kidney Disease

Research has shown that the gut microbiome, which consists of trillions of bacteria and other microorganisms, plays an essential role in our overall health. In individuals with CKD, the gut microbiome may become imbalanced, leading to a condition called gut dysbiosis. This imbalance can contribute to increased inflammation, a weakened immune system, and reduced nutrient absorption – all factors that can negatively impact kidney function.

Moreover, an imbalanced gut microbiome can lead to the production of harmful toxins such as uremic toxins, which can further damage the kidneys. Thus, promoting a healthy gut microbiome is essential for managing CKD and maintaining overall well-being.

Probiotics and Prebiotics for Kidney Patients

Probiotics are live microorganisms, usually bacteria or

yeast, that can help improve gut health by maintaining or restoring the balance of beneficial bacteria in the gut. Renadyl (https://go.DadviceTV.com/Renadyl), a unique blend of beneficial probiotics and prebiotics designed specifically for kidney patients, is often recommended by renal dietitians and healthcare teams to support gut health in individuals with CKD. Renadyl has been part of my healthy lifestyle since shortly after being diagnosed.

Prebiotics, on the other hand, are non-digestible fibers that serve as food for the beneficial bacteria in your gut. They stimulate the growth and activity of these bacteria, thereby promoting a balanced gut microbiome.

Incorporating Gut-Friendly Foods into Your Diet

A well-rounded, kidney-friendly diet should include a variety of gut-friendly foods that are rich in probiotics and prebiotics. Here are some suggestions for incorporating these foods into your diet:

1. Probiotic-rich foods: Incorporate probiotic-rich foods such as yogurt, kefir, and fermented vegetables (e.g., sauerkraut, kimchi) into your diet. Be sure to choose low-sodium and low-phosphorus options, as some fermented foods can be high in these minerals.

2. Prebiotic-rich foods: Include prebiotic-rich foods like onions, garlic, leeks, asparagus, and whole grains in your diet. These foods help nourish the beneficial bacteria in your gut and promote a balanced gut microbiome.

3. Fruits and vegetables: Aim for a diet rich in plant-based foods, including a variety of colorful fruits and vegetables. These foods are high in fiber and antioxidants, which can help support gut health and reduce inflammation.

4. Whole grains: Choose whole grains over refined grains, as they are higher in fiber and can help promote a healthy gut microbiome. Opt for kidney-friendly whole grains like quinoa, barley, and bulgur.

5. Limit processed foods: Processed foods can be high in salt, sugar, and unhealthy fats, which can negatively impact gut health. Focus on consuming whole, minimally processed foods as much as possible.

6. Stay hydrated: Drinking an adequate amount of water is essential for maintaining gut health. Be sure to discuss your individual fluid intake needs with your healthcare team, as some individuals with CKD may need to limit their fluid consumption.

Research Supporting the Role of Gut Health in CKD

Several studies have highlighted the importance of gut health in individuals with CKD. Research has shown that an imbalanced gut microbiome can contribute to inflammation, oxidative stress, and the production of harmful toxins, all of which can negatively affect kidney function. Furthermore, studies have demonstrated that interventions targeting gut health, such as the use of probiotics and prebiotics, can help improve clinical outcomes in CKD patients.

For instance, a study published in the Journal of Renal Nutrition found that supplementation with probiotics and prebiotics could help reduce inflammation and oxidative stress in individuals with CKD, which are known contributors to kidney damage. Additionally, a review published in the journal Nutrients concluded that interventions targeting the gut microbiome, including dietary modifications and the use of probiotics, may help slow the progression of CKD and improve overall health in affected individuals.

While more research is needed to fully understand the relationship between gut health and kidney disease, the existing evidence suggests that maintaining a healthy gut microbiome is an essential component of CKD management.

Promoting gut health is crucial for individuals with chronic kidney disease, as a healthy gut microbiome can positively influence immune function, metabolism, and nutrient absorption, all of which can impact kidney function. By incorporating gut-friendly foods into your diet, such as probiotics, prebiotics, fruits, vegetables, and whole grains, you can support a balanced gut microbiome and help slow the progression of CKD.

THE KIDNEY DIET: FOODS TO WATCH

Embarking on a kidney-friendly diet can be a significant lifestyle change, but it's crucial for maintaining optimal kidney health. This chapter will highlight common foods that kidney patients should monitor and limit in their daily meals without outrightly discouraging their consumption. Remember, moderation is key, and it's essential to consult your healthcare provider or a renal dietitian to develop a personalized dietary plan.

Highly Processed Foods: Processed foods often contain high amounts of sodium, unhealthy fats, and added sugars, which can strain your kidneys. Instead, opt for whole, unprocessed foods to ensure a nutrient-dense, kidney-friendly diet.

High Sodium Foods: Excess sodium intake can cause fluid retention and increase blood pressure, putting additional stress on your kidneys. Monitor your consumption of high-sodium foods, such as canned soups, processed meats, fast food, and salty snacks. Instead, choose low-sodium alternatives and use herbs and spices for flavoring.

Foods High in Potassium: While potassium is vital for maintaining a healthy heart rhythm, excessive amounts can be dangerous for kidney patients. Limit high-potassium foods like bananas, avocados, oranges, potatoes, tomatoes, and spinach. Consult your healthcare provider for personalized potassium intake recommendations.

Foods Rich in Phosphorus: High phosphorus levels can lead

to weak bones and kidney damage. Kidney patients should be cautious about their intake of phosphorus-rich foods such as dairy products, beans, lentils, nuts, and seeds. Opt for lower phosphorus alternatives and prioritize portion control.

Animal Proteins: Although protein is an essential nutrient, excessive animal protein consumption can burden the kidneys. Focus on lean protein sources, such as fish and poultry, and consider incorporating plant-based proteins like legumes and tofu for better kidney health.

Refined Carbohydrates: Foods like white bread, pasta, and pastries contain refined carbohydrates that can cause blood sugar fluctuations and stress the kidneys. Opt for whole grains like brown rice, quinoa, and whole-wheat bread for a healthier choice.

Sugary Beverages: Soda, fruit juice, and energy drinks are high in sugar and can contribute to weight gain, diabetes, and kidney damage. Choose water, herbal tea, or sugar-free beverages to stay hydrated without taxing your kidneys.

Alcohol: Excessive alcohol consumption can lead to high blood pressure, liver damage, and kidney problems. Limit your alcohol intake and focus on hydrating with water and other non-alcoholic beverages.

"IS THIS FOOD OKAY FOR ME?" - NAVIGATING DIETARY CHOICES

Navigating the world of dietary choices when living with kidney disease can be challenging. A common question that arises is, "Is this food okay for me?" It's normal to be concerned about how your diet may affect your kidney health, particularly with the vast amount of information available. This chapter aims to guide you through the key principles of a kidney-friendly diet and provide practical tips on enjoying a wide variety of foods without compromising your kidney health.

Foundational Principles of a Kidney-Friendly Diet

Before delving into specific food choices, it's important to grasp the core principles of a kidney-friendly diet. The main objectives of this diet include:

- Protecting kidney function and preventing further damage.
- Managing symptoms and complications associated with kidney disease.
- Supporting overall health and well-being.

To achieve these objectives, a kidney-friendly diet generally emphasizes:

- Reducing sodium intake to help control blood pressure and prevent fluid retention.
- Maintaining healthy potassium levels to ensure a proper balance of electrolytes in the body.
- Regulating phosphorus intake to prevent high levels in the blood, which can lead to bone and heart issues.
- Watching protein consumption to decrease the

workload on the kidneys while ensuring sufficient nutrition.

• Balancing caloric intake to maintain a healthy weight and prevent malnutrition.

• Ensuring adequate intake of essential vitamins and minerals.

The Key to Variety: Portion Control is Essential

The secret to enjoying an array of foods while adhering to a kidney-friendly diet is embracing moderation. Instead of strictly avoiding certain foods, concentrate on portion control and balance. Almost any food can be incorporated into a heart-healthy, kidney-friendly diet when consumed in moderation and as part of a balanced meal plan.

For instance, enjoying a slice of cake and a scoop of ice cream at a celebration is perfectly acceptable, as long as you account for the additional sugar, sodium, and other nutrients in your overall meal plan. This may mean consuming fewer sugary foods during the rest of the day or making adjustments to your meal plan in the days leading up to the event.

Tips for Including a Broad Range of Foods in Your Diet

Plan Your Meals: Meal planning allows you to create a balanced meal plan that takes into account the nutrients in various foods. This ensures that you can enjoy a wide range of foods while adhering to your dietary guidelines.

Master Food Label Reading: Knowing how to read food labels is vital for managing your kidney-friendly diet. Get acquainted with the key nutrients to monitor (sodium, potassium, phosphorus, protein, and calories) and use this information to make informed choices about the foods you eat.

Opt for Nutrient-Rich Foods: Choose nutrient-rich foods that offer essential vitamins and minerals without excessive amounts of sodium, potassium, or phosphorus. This enables you to obtain the most nutritional value from the foods you eat while minimizing the impact on your kidneys.

Practice Portion Control: Be mindful of portion sizes when savoring your favorite foods. Overindulging in any food can lead to an imbalance in your diet and negatively affect your kidney health. Stick to recommended serving sizes and savor each bite.

Make Healthy Food Swaps: Look for ways to make healthier substitutions in your favorite recipes. This could involve swapping high-sodium ingredients for low-sodium alternatives, using herbs and spices instead of salt to flavor your food, or choosing whole grains over refined grains to increase fiber intake.

Enjoy Treats in Moderation: It's important to strike a balance between maintaining a kidney-friendly diet and indulging in the occasional treat. Enjoying a small portion of your favorite dessert or snack now and then can make your meal plan more enjoyable and sustainable. Remember to account for these treats in your overall nutrient intake and make adjustments as necessary.

Communicate with Your Healthcare Team: Keep your healthcare team informed about your dietary choices and any changes you make to your meal plan. They can provide personalized guidance and support to help you maintain a balanced, kidney-friendly diet while enjoying a diverse range of foods.

Listen to Your Body: Pay attention to how your body responds to different foods and make adjustments as needed. If you notice changes in your symptoms or lab results, discuss these with your healthcare team and consider making modifications to your diet.

Educate Yourself: The more you know about kidney disease and nutrition, the better equipped you will be to make informed decisions about your diet. Stay up-to-date on the latest research and dietary recommendations, and don't hesitate to ask your healthcare team for clarification or guidance.

By understanding the fundamentals of a kidney-friendly diet and applying practical strategies, you can confidently navigate your dietary choices and enjoy a wide variety of foods that support your kidney health.

STARFRUIT AND CKD - A DANGEROUS COMBINATION

While a kidney-friendly diet often allows for the inclusion of various fruits and vegetables, there are some exceptions that individuals with kidney disease should be aware of. Starfruit, also known as carambola, is one such exception. This tropical fruit, with its unique shape and sweet, tangy flavor, can pose a severe risk to those with compromised kidney function. In this chapter, we will explore the dangers associated with consuming starfruit for individuals with kidney disease and why it is best to leave this fruit out of a kidney-friendly diet.

The Hidden Dangers of Starfruit for Kidney Patients

At first glance, starfruit might seem like a healthy, nutritious option for individuals with kidney disease. However, the fruit contains a neurotoxin called caramboxin, which is harmful to those with impaired kidney function. In healthy individuals, the kidneys efficiently filter caramboxin from the bloodstream, and the toxin is excreted through urine without any adverse effects.

Unfortunately, in individuals with kidney disease, the kidneys' ability to filter and eliminate caramboxin is significantly reduced or impaired. As a result, the toxin accumulates in the bloodstream, leading to a series of potentially life-threatening neurological symptoms and complications.

Symptoms of Starfruit Toxicity

The symptoms of starfruit toxicity can range from mild to severe, depending on the extent of kidney dysfunction and the amount of starfruit consumed. Some common symptoms associated with starfruit toxicity include:

- Confusion
- Hiccups
- Seizures
- Vomiting
- Weakness
- Altered mental status

In extreme cases, starfruit toxicity can lead to coma and even death. The severity of symptoms and the rapidity of their onset can vary among individuals, making it crucial for those with kidney disease to avoid starfruit consumption entirely.

Managing the Risk: Avoiding Starfruit in a Kidney-Friendly Diet

Given the potential dangers associated with starfruit consumption for individuals with kidney disease, it is essential to avoid this fruit in a kidney-friendly diet. Here are some tips to help you manage the risk:

1. Be aware of the dangers: Educate yourself about the risks associated with starfruit consumption and inform your family members, friends, and caregivers. This awareness can help prevent accidental ingestion of starfruit.

2. Read food labels: While starfruit is not a common ingredient in processed foods, it's essential to read food labels and be cautious of any unfamiliar

ingredients.

3. Be cautious when dining out: If you're eating out or attending social events, be aware of dishes that might contain starfruit. Don't hesitate to ask questions about the ingredients in your meal and inform your server or host about your dietary restrictions.

4. Choose alternative fruits: There are many other kidney-friendly fruits available that can provide essential nutrients without posing a risk to your health. Some examples include apples, berries, cherries, grapes, and pineapple. Consult your healthcare team or dietitian for personalized recommendations on fruit intake.

5. Consult with a dietitian: A registered dietitian specializing in kidney disease can help you develop a meal plan that meets your nutritional needs while avoiding starfruit and other potential risks.

6. Inform your healthcare team: Make sure your healthcare team is aware of your dietary choices and any changes you make to your meal plan. They can provide additional guidance and support to help you maintain a safe, balanced, kidney-friendly diet.

THE BEST DIET FOR CKD

The best diet for kidney disease is one that addresses the unique nutritional needs of each individual while also promoting overall health and well-being. A heart-healthy, individualized diet rich in plant-based foods is the key to managing kidney disease and slowing its progression. In this chapter, we will discuss the importance of working with a dietitian to customize a kidney-friendly diet, the benefits of plant-based eating, and the suitability of the DASH diet for many kidney patients.

The Importance of a Heart-Healthy, Individualized Diet

A well-rounded, heart-healthy diet is of paramount importance in managing kidney disease and preserving overall health. It is vital to understand that one-size-fits-all diets or food lists **do not work**. Each person's dietary requirements must be individualized and adjusted based on their health, existing conditions such as diabetes or high blood pressure, their lifestyle, activity level, and lab results. By emphasizing foods that promote cardiovascular health and tailoring the diet to meet each individual's unique needs, it becomes possible to slow the progression of kidney disease and enhance the quality of life.

Working with a Dietitian for a Customized Kidney-Friendly Diet

As a kidney health coach, I cannot stress enough the

importance of working closely with a dietitian to develop a personalized meal plan. A dietitian specializes in understanding the complex nutritional requirements of individuals with kidney disease and can provide the education and tools necessary to make confident, healthy eating choices. Some benefits of working with a dietitian include:

Personalized guidance: A dietitian can assess your unique nutritional needs based on factors such as age, weight, lifestyle, and stage of kidney disease. This personalized approach ensures that your diet is tailored to meet your specific requirements.

Ongoing support: As your kidney function changes, so too will your dietary needs. A dietitian can provide ongoing support and adjustments to your meal plan to ensure that it remains effective and appropriate for your changing needs.

Education: A dietitian can teach you about the relationship between nutrition and kidney health, helping you to make informed decisions about the foods you consume.

Confidence: By working with a dietitian, you can feel confident in your ability to make healthy eating choices that support your kidney health and overall well-being.

The Benefits of Plant-Based Eating for Kidney Patients

A diet rich in plant-based foods offers numerous benefits for individuals with kidney disease. Plant-based foods are naturally low in sodium, potassium, and phosphorus, making them an ideal choice for a kidney-friendly diet. Some additional benefits of plant-based eating include:

Improved cardiovascular health: A plant-based diet can help lower blood pressure, cholesterol levels, and reduce the risk of heart disease, which is especially important for kidney patients.

Better blood sugar control: Plant-based foods are rich in fiber and low in added sugars, which can help stabilize blood sugar levels and manage diabetes, a common risk factor for kidney disease.

Reduced inflammation: A diet rich in plant-based foods can help reduce inflammation in the body, which is associated with kidney disease progression.

Enhanced gut health: Plant-based foods, particularly those high in fiber, can improve gut health and promote a healthy balance of gut bacteria, which can be beneficial for individuals with kidney disease.

The DASH Diet: A Common Option for Kidney Patients

The DASH (Dietary Approaches to Stop Hypertension) diet is a popular heart-healthy eating plan that can be adapted for kidney patients. This diet emphasizes the consumption of fruits, vegetables, whole grains, lean proteins, and low-fat dairy products while limiting sodium, saturated fat, and added sugars. Some benefits of the DASH diet for kidney patients include:

1. **Improved blood pressure control**: The DASH diet is designed to help lower blood pressure, which is crucial for managing kidney disease and preventing further kidney damage.

2. **Balanced nutrient intake**: The DASH diet promotes a balanced intake of essential nutrients while also helping individuals manage their sodium, potassium, and phosphorus levels, which is vital for maintaining kidney health.

3. **Flexibility**: The DASH diet can be easily adapted to accommodate individual dietary preferences and restrictions, making it a versatile option for kidney patients.

4. **Evidence-based**: The DASH diet is supported by extensive research and has been shown to improve

cardiovascular health and reduce the risk of chronic diseases, including kidney disease.

Other Popular Diets for Kidney Patients

While the DASH diet is a popular choice for kidney patients, there are other dietary approaches that can also help manage kidney disease and its complications. Below, we explore some of these diets and the research supporting their use in kidney patients.

1. Mediterranean Diet

The Mediterranean diet is rich in fruits, vegetables, whole grains, legumes, nuts, and olive oil, with moderate amounts of fish, poultry, and dairy products. It emphasizes the consumption of healthy fats, such as monounsaturated and polyunsaturated fats, while limiting the intake of saturated fats and trans fats. The Mediterranean diet is known for its numerous health benefits, including improved cardiovascular health, reduced risk of chronic diseases, and weight management.

A study published in the Clinical Journal of the American Society of Nephrology found that adherence to a Mediterranean-style diet was associated with a lower risk of developing chronic kidney disease (CKD) and a slower decline in kidney function among those with existing CKD (Gutiérrez et al., 2013).

2. Plant-Based Diet

A plant-based diet focuses on consuming whole, minimally processed plant foods, such as fruits, vegetables, whole grains, legumes, nuts, and seeds. This diet is typically low in sodium, saturated fat, and cholesterol, and rich in fiber, antioxidants, and essential nutrients. A plant-based diet can be tailored to include varying amounts of animal products, depending on individual preferences and needs.

A study in the Journal of Renal Nutrition found that

CKD patients who followed a plant-based diet experienced improvements in blood pressure, cholesterol, and kidney function, as well as a reduced risk of cardiovascular events and mortality (Chauveau et al., 2013).

3. Low-Protein Diet

A low-protein diet involves restricting the intake of dietary protein to help minimize the workload on the kidneys and reduce the production of waste products. This diet may be recommended for patients with advanced kidney disease or those at risk of rapid progression. Beware, a low-protein diet can be dangerous for some kidney patients. It's essential to work closely with a dietitian to ensure that adequate nutrition is maintained while on a low-protein diet.

A systematic review and meta-analysis published in the American Journal of Kidney Diseases found that low-protein diets can help slow the progression of CKD, particularly in patients with diabetes or at high risk of kidney failure (Menon et al., 2009).

The best diet for kidney disease is a heart-healthy, individualized plan that prioritizes plant-based foods and takes into account each individual's unique needs. Working with a dietitian to create a customized meal plan is crucial for managing kidney disease and slowing its progression. The DASH diet is a popular, evidence-based option that can be adapted for kidney patients, providing a well-balanced, flexible approach to eating that promotes overall health and well-being.

As a kidney health coach, I strongly encourage kidney patients to **seek the guidance of a dietitian**. With their expertise and support, you can develop the skills and knowledge necessary to make confident, healthy eating choices that will benefit your kidney health.

PLANT-BASED IS NOT VEGETARIAN

In the world of kidney health, the term "plant-based diet" often conjures up images of strict vegetarian or vegan lifestyles. However, this doesn't have to be the case! A plant-based diet simply means incorporating more plant-based foods into your meals while still enjoying animal products in moderation. This chapter aims to show you the bright side of plant-based eating and how it can benefit your kidney health, without depriving you of your favorite non-vegetarian dishes.

One of the primary benefits of a plant-based diet is the increased fiber intake. Fruits, vegetables, whole grains, and legumes are rich in dietary fiber, which helps maintain bowel health, lower cholesterol levels, and keep blood sugar levels stable. A diet rich in fiber has also been linked to a reduced risk of heart disease, obesity, and certain types of cancer. By increasing your plant-based food consumption, you'll be doing your kidneys and overall health a huge favor!

Now, let's talk about incorporating animal products in a healthy, plant-based diet. You can absolutely include eggs, chicken, turkey, and other animal-based products in your meals. The key is to strike a balance between plant-based foods and animal products, using portion control to ensure you're getting the right nutrients without overloading on protein, sodium, or other potentially harmful components. For instance, you can have a colorful salad filled with fresh veggies, beans, and avocado, topped with a small portion of grilled chicken or a boiled egg.

Remember that a plant-based diet doesn't mean you have to give up the foods you love. Instead, it's about embracing variety and adding more plant-based options to your plate. Get creative with your meal planning and try new recipes that incorporate a mix of plant-based and animal-based ingredients. The more you experiment with different food combinations, cooking methods, and seasonings, the more you'll discover exciting ways to enjoy a healthy, kidney-friendly diet.

Adopting a plant-based diet is a fantastic way to improve your kidney health without feeling restricted or deprived. By focusing on balance and variety, you can enjoy a diverse range of foods that are both delicious and beneficial for your overall well-being. So, go ahead and make plants the star of your plate, but remember that a little bit of animal-based goodness can still have a place in your kidney-friendly diet.

Sample of a one-day meal plan

Breakfast:

- 1 cup cooked oatmeal, topped with a small handful of blueberries and a drizzle of honey
- 1 slice of whole-grain toast with 1 tablespoon of almond butter
- 8 oz unsweetened almond milk
- 1 cup of black coffee or herbal tea (optional)

Morning Snack:

- 1 small apple, sliced
- 1 oz of low-sodium, kidney-friendly cheese

Lunch:

- 2 cups mixed greens salad with cherry tomatoes, cucumber, and red bell pepper slices
- 3 oz grilled chicken breast or tofu (for a vegetarian

option)
- 1/4 cup cooked quinoa or brown rice
- 1 tablespoon of low-sodium vinaigrette dressing

Afternoon Snack:
- 1/2 cup baby carrots
- 2 tablespoons of hummus

Dinner:
- 1 cup cooked whole wheat pasta, tossed with 1/2 cup kidney-friendly marinara sauce (low-sodium)
- 1/2 cup steamed green beans or zucchini
- 2 oz baked or grilled salmon, seasoned with fresh herbs and lemon juice
- 1 small whole-grain dinner roll with 1 teaspoon of unsalted butter

Evening Snack:
- 1/2 cup of mixed fresh fruit salad (limit high-potassium fruits like bananas, oranges, and kiwi if you are on a potassium restriction)

Remember to consult with your healthcare team and renal dietitian before making any significant changes to your diet. They can help tailor a meal plan that specifically meets your individual needs and restrictions based on your kidney function and other health factors.

MULTIVITAMINS FOR CKD PATIENTS

As kidney function declines, the body's ability to properly absorb and utilize essential vitamins and minerals may become impaired. This can lead to deficiencies that negatively impact overall health and well-being. For individuals with CKD, it is crucial to ensure adequate intake of essential nutrients through a balanced diet and, in some cases, supplementation with specialized multivitamins. In this chapter, we will discuss the importance of multivitamins for CKD patients, the unique needs and challenges they face, and the role of ProRenal+D, a renal dietitian-recommended multivitamin I take, in supporting kidney health.

The Importance of Multivitamins for CKD Patients

As kidney function declines, individuals with CKD may experience alterations in their nutritional status. Some common challenges faced by CKD patients include:

1. Altered appetite and dietary restrictions: CKD patients may experience a reduced appetite, making it difficult to consume enough calories and nutrients. Additionally, dietary restrictions imposed to manage CKD, such as limiting sodium, potassium, and phosphorus, can further compound the challenge of obtaining essential nutrients.

2. Impaired absorption and utilization: CKD can

impair the absorption and utilization of certain nutrients, such as vitamin D, which plays a critical role in bone health and immune function. Moreover, metabolic acidosis, a common complication of CKD, can lead to the loss of important nutrients like bicarbonate, further exacerbating nutritional imbalances.

3. Increased nutrient losses: CKD patients may lose essential nutrients through dialysis or impaired kidney function. Dialysis, in particular, can cause the removal of water-soluble vitamins, such as vitamin C and B-complex vitamins, from the body.

4. Drug-nutrient interactions: Medications commonly prescribed for CKD patients, such as phosphate binders and diuretics, can interfere with the absorption and metabolism of certain nutrients, leading to deficiencies.

Given these challenges, it is crucial for CKD patients to work closely with their healthcare team, including a renal dietitian, to identify potential nutrient deficiencies and develop a personalized plan for supplementation with multivitamins that are specifically formulated to address their unique needs.

The Role of ProRenal+D in Supporting Kidney Health

ProRenal+D (MyProRenal.com) is a renal dietitian-recommended multivitamin designed specifically for individuals with CKD. This unique formulation takes into account the nutritional needs and challenges faced by CKD patients and provides targeted support for kidney health. Some key features of ProRenal+D include:

1. Tailored nutrient profile: ProRenal+D contains a blend of essential vitamins and minerals that are carefully selected to meet the specific needs of CKD

patients. These nutrients are provided in amounts that are safe and effective for individuals with impaired kidney function, avoiding the risk of overloading the kidneys with excessive nutrients.

2. Vitamin D support: Vitamin D deficiency is common in CKD patients due to impaired activation of the vitamin by the kidneys. ProRenal+D contains cholecalciferol (vitamin D3), the preferred form of vitamin D for individuals with CKD, to support bone health, immune function, and overall well-being.

3. B-complex vitamins: B-complex vitamins, including B1 (thiamine), B2 (riboflavin), B3 (niacin), B6 (pyridoxine), B9 (folic acid), and B12 (cobalamin), play a critical role in energy production, red blood cell formation, and nerve function. ProRenal+D provides these essential nutrients in safe amounts to help support the unique needs of CKD patients.

4. Antioxidant support: Oxidative stress is a significant factor in the progression of CKD, and individuals with this condition may benefit from increased antioxidant support. ProRenal+D contains a blend of antioxidants, including vitamins C and E, which help neutralize harmful free radicals and protect cells from oxidative damage.

5. Mineral balance: CKD patients often need to monitor and limit their intake of certain minerals, such as potassium and phosphorus. ProRenal+D is formulated without these minerals, ensuring that individuals with CKD can safely take this multivitamin without exacerbating mineral imbalances.

6. Enhanced bioavailability: The nutrients in ProRenal +D are provided in forms that are easily absorbed and utilized by the body, ensuring optimal benefit for individuals with CKD.

When to Consider a Renal Multivitamin

It is essential for individuals with CKD to work closely with their healthcare team, including a renal dietitian, to assess their nutritional needs and determine whether supplementation with a multivitamin is appropriate. Factors that may indicate a need for supplementation include:

- Poor dietary intake or adherence to dietary restrictions
- Persistent nutrient deficiencies identified through blood tests
- Significant weight loss or muscle wasting
- Dialysis treatment, which can lead to increased nutrient losses

Before starting any supplement regimen, it is crucial to discuss your specific needs and goals with your healthcare team to ensure that the chosen product is safe, effective, and appropriate for your unique situation.

Tips for Incorporating a Multivitamin into Your Daily Routine

Take the multivitamin as directed by your healthcare team, typically once daily with a meal to optimize absorption and minimize the risk of gastrointestinal side effects.

Monitor your nutrient levels through regular blood tests and follow-up appointments with your healthcare team to ensure that your supplementation regimen is meeting your needs and not causing any adverse effects.

Remember that multivitamins are meant to complement, not replace, a balanced diet. Continue to prioritize a nutrient-dense, kidney-friendly diet that includes a variety of whole, minimally processed foods.

Keep an open line of communication with your healthcare team and notify them of any changes in your symptoms, medications, or overall health status, as these factors may impact your nutritional needs and supplementation regimen.

7-DAY MEAL PLAN EXAMPLE (NO RESTRICTIONS)

The following is one of my actual 7-day meal plans that I used at Stage 3 with no diet restrictions. This was created specifically for me and serves as an example.

Day 1:

- Breakfast: Overnight oats with almond milk, chia seeds, and blueberries
- Lunch: Chickpea salad with cherry tomatoes, cucumber, red onion, and lemon-tahini dressing
- Dinner: Grilled chicken breast with quinoa and roasted Brussels sprouts
- Snack: Apple slices with almond butter

Day 2:

- Breakfast: Green smoothie with spinach, banana, flaxseeds, and unsweetened almond milk
- Lunch: Lentil soup with whole-grain bread and a side salad
- Dinner: Baked salmon with brown rice and steamed green beans
- Snack: Fresh fruit salad

Day 3:

- Breakfast: Egg scramble with spinach, tomatoes, and avocado
- Lunch: Buddha bowl with quinoa, roasted sweet potatoes, black beans, and avocado-lime dressing
- Dinner: Vegetable stir-fry with tofu and brown rice
- Snack: Hummus and raw veggie sticks

Day 4:

- Breakfast: Greek yogurt with mixed berries and a sprinkle of chopped nuts
- Lunch: Grilled chicken and vegetable wrap with whole-grain tortilla and a side of mixed greens
- Dinner: Eggplant Parmesan with a side of whole-grain pasta and steamed broccoli
- Snack: Rice cake with avocado and cherry tomatoes

Day 5:

- Breakfast: Chia seed pudding with sliced almonds and honey
- Lunch: Mediterranean quinoa salad with olives, feta cheese, and lemon-olive oil dressing
- Dinner: Roasted vegetable and chickpea curry with basmati rice
- Snack: Yogurt with granola and a drizzle of honey

Day 6:

- Breakfast: Smoothie bowl with banana, spinach, unsweetened almond milk, and toppings of choice (e.g., nuts, seeds, coconut flakes)
- Lunch: Grilled portobello mushroom burger with a whole-grain bun and a side of mixed greens
- Dinner: Baked chicken with lemon and garlic, served

with roasted asparagus and couscous
- Snack: Sliced cucumber and carrot sticks with a Greek yogurt-based dip

Day 7:

- Breakfast: Whole-grain toast with avocado, cherry tomatoes, and a poached egg
- Lunch: Lentil and vegetable-stuffed bell peppers with a side of mixed greens
- Dinner: Cauliflower rice stir-fry with mixed vegetables, cashews, and a soy-free, low-sodium sauce
- Snack: Fresh fruit smoothie with unsweetened almond milk

Please note that this meal plan is a general guide and may not be suitable for everyone. Consult a renal dietitian to create a personalized meal plan tailored to your specific needs and preferences.

7-DAY MEAL PLAN EXAMPLE (POTASSIUM RESTRICTION)

The following is one of my actual 7-day meal plans that I used at Stage 4 with a 2700mg daily potassium restriction. This was created specifically for me and serves as an example.

Day 1:

- Breakfast: Cream of wheat with almond milk, a drizzle of honey, and blueberries
- Lunch: Egg salad sandwich on whole-grain bread with lettuce and cucumber
- Dinner: Baked lemon-herb chicken with rice and green beans
- Snack: Apple slices with a tablespoon of peanut butter

Day 2:

- Breakfast: Smoothie with strawberries, pineapple, and unsweetened almond milk
- Lunch: Grilled chicken Caesar salad with low-potassium dressing and whole-grain croutons
- Dinner: Vegetable stir-fry with chicken, bamboo shoots, and white rice

- Snack: Rice cakes with cream cheese and cucumber slices

Day 3:

- Breakfast: English muffin with scrambled eggs, tomato, and lettuce
- Lunch: Chickpea and cucumber salad with red onion, cherry tomatoes, and a lemon-tahini dressing
- Dinner: Baked salmon with couscous and steamed zucchini
- Snack: Low-potassium fruit salad (e.g., apple, grapes, pineapple)

Day 4:

- Breakfast: Greek yogurt with blueberries and a tablespoon of honey
- Lunch: Tuna salad wrap with lettuce, cucumber, and whole-grain tortilla
- Dinner: Chicken and vegetable kebabs with rice and a side of mixed greens
- Snack: Carrot and celery sticks with a low-potassium dip

Day 5:

- Breakfast: Toast with almond butter and sliced strawberries
- Lunch: Garden salad with grilled chicken, cucumber, and a low-potassium dressing
- Dinner: Spaghetti squash with marinara sauce and a side of steamed green beans
- Snack: Crackers with cream cheese and sliced cucumber

Day 6:

- Breakfast: Oatmeal with almond milk, a drizzle of

honey, and chopped apple

- Lunch: Turkey and cheese sandwich on whole-grain bread with lettuce and sliced cucumber
- Dinner: Baked chicken with lemon and garlic, served with mashed cauliflower and steamed zucchini
- Snack: A small portion of unsalted nuts and dried cranberries

Day 7:

- Breakfast: Pancakes made with almond flour, topped with blueberries and a drizzle of maple syrup
- Lunch: Quinoa salad with cherry tomatoes, cucumber, and red onion, dressed with a low-potassium vinaigrette
- Dinner: Veggie and chicken stir-fry with low-sodium soy sauce and white rice
- Snack: Low-potassium fruit smoothie made with pineapple, strawberries, and unsweetened almond milk

Please note that this meal plan is a general guide and may not be suitable for everyone. Consult a renal dietitian to create a personalized meal plan tailored to your specific needs and preferences. Keep in mind that individual potassium restrictions may vary, so it's important to track your intake and adjust accordingly.

AVOIDING COMMON DIET MISTAKES

Navigating a kidney-friendly diet can be challenging, and it's natural to make mistakes along the way. In this chapter, we'll discuss some common diet mistakes kidney patients make and offer guidance on how to avoid them. Our goal is to help you make informed choices about your diet to better manage your kidney disease and improve your overall health.

Over-Restricting and Eliminating Foods Unnecessarily

Many kidney patients feel overwhelmed by dietary restrictions and may over-restrict their diet, eliminating foods that are not necessarily harmful. This can lead to an unbalanced and nutritionally inadequate diet, depriving your body of essential nutrients. Instead of eliminating entire food groups, focus on portion control and moderation. Work with a renal dietitian to create a personalized meal plan that meets your nutritional needs and accommodates your taste preferences.

Not Individualizing Your Diet Based on Your Health and Lab Results

Kidney disease affects everyone differently, and a one-size-fits-all approach to diet is not ideal. It's essential to tailor your diet based on your specific health needs and lab results. Factors such as your stage of kidney disease, other medical conditions, and nutrient levels should all be considered when creating your meal plan. Collaborate with your healthcare team and renal dietitian to develop a customized dietary strategy that supports your unique situation.

Relying on Supplements Instead of Food

While supplements can be helpful in some cases, they should not replace a balanced diet. Over-reliance on supplements can lead to nutrient imbalances and other health problems. Focus on obtaining nutrients from whole foods, and use supplements only as directed by your healthcare team. Remember that supplements should complement, not substitute, a well-rounded diet.

Following Diet Advice from Random Strangers on Social Media Sites

Social media can be a valuable source of information and support for kidney patients. However, it's crucial to be cautious about the advice you encounter online. Some individuals may share misleading or even harmful recommendations based on their own experiences or beliefs. Always consult your healthcare team and renal dietitian before making significant changes to your diet, and be skeptical of advice that seems too good to be true or contradicts professional guidance.

Not Reading Food Labels

Understanding what you're eating is crucial for managing your kidney-friendly diet. Many packaged foods contain hidden additives, preservatives, and excess sodium, which can negatively impact your kidney health. Make it a habit to read food labels and choose products with fewer ingredients and less processed components. Prioritize consuming real, whole foods to support your nutritional needs and overall health.

Not Experimenting with Food Combinations, Cooking Methods, and Seasonings

A common pitfall for kidney patients is becoming stuck in a dietary rut, eating the same foods and dishes repeatedly. This can lead to boredom and frustration, making it challenging to stick to a kidney-friendly diet. To add variety and excitement to your meals, experiment with different food combinations, cooking methods, and seasonings. Get creative in the kitchen and explore new recipes and flavors that align with your dietary restrictions.

Managing your diet as a kidney patient can be complex, but it's an essential aspect of managing your kidney disease. By avoiding these common mistakes and working closely with your healthcare team, you can develop a personalized dietary strategy that supports your overall health and well-being. Remember, every journey has its challenges, but with patience, persistence, and a caring support system, you can confidently navigate your kidney-friendly diet.

EXERCISE AND PHYSICAL ACTIVITY

Exercise and physical activity play a crucial role in maintaining overall health and well-being, especially for individuals with chronic kidney disease (CKD). Engaging in regular exercise can offer numerous benefits, including improved cardiovascular health, better management of symptoms and complications, and enhanced quality of life. This chapter will discuss the benefits of exercise, guidelines and recommendations for those with CKD, considerations for different stages of CKD, tips for incorporating exercise into your life, and recommended exercises for those with limited mobility.

Benefits of Exercise for Kidney Patients

Regular exercise offers several benefits for kidney patients, including:

1. Improved cardiovascular health: Exercise helps lower blood pressure, reduce cholesterol levels, and maintain a healthy weight, reducing the risk of heart disease and stroke.

2. Better blood sugar control: Physical activity helps manage blood glucose levels, which is essential for people with diabetes, a common cause of CKD.

3. Enhanced muscle strength and endurance: Exercise helps maintain and improve muscle strength, enabling kidney patients to perform daily activities with ease.

4. Increased energy levels: Regular physical activity can help combat fatigue and increase overall energy levels.

5. Improved mental well-being: Exercise can reduce stress, anxiety, and depression, improving emotional well-being and quality of life.

Guidelines and Recommendations for CKD Patients

It's essential to consult with your healthcare team before starting an exercise program, as they can provide personalized recommendations based on your current health status, stage of kidney disease, and other factors. General guidelines for CKD patients include:

1. Aim for at least 150 minutes of moderate-intensity aerobic exercise per week, spread over at least three days, with no more than two consecutive days without exercise.

2. Include muscle-strengthening activities, such as resistance training, at least two days per week.

3. Perform flexibility exercises, such as stretching, yoga, or tai chi, to maintain joint mobility and prevent injury.

4. Incorporate balance exercises, particularly for older adults or those at risk of falls.

Types of Exercise for CKD Patients

1. Aerobic exercise: Activities such as walking, cycling, swimming, or dancing, which increase heart rate and improve cardiovascular fitness.

2. Resistance training: Exercises using body weight, resistance bands, or weights to strengthen muscles and improve overall strength.

3. Flexibility exercises: Stretching, yoga, or pilates, which improve joint mobility and prevent injury.

4. Balance exercises: Activities such as standing on one leg, heel-to-toe walking, or tai chi, which enhance balance and reduce the risk of falls.

Considerations for Different Stages of CKD

As kidney function declines, certain adjustments to your exercise routine may be necessary. Always consult your healthcare team for personalized recommendations based on your specific needs.

Early stages of CKD (stages 1-3): At this stage, patients can usually engage in regular exercise routines with few modifications.

Advanced stages of CKD (stages 4-5): Patients in these stages may need to modify their exercise intensity and duration to accommodate reduced kidney function and potential complications.

Dialysis patients: Those on dialysis may need to adjust their exercise schedule around treatment sessions and manage fluid intake during exercise.

Tips for Incorporating Exercise into Your Life

1. Start gradually: Begin with low-intensity activities and gradually increase intensity and duration as your fitness improves.

2. Set realistic goals: Establish achievable and measurable goals to track your progress and stay motivated.

3. Find activities you enjoy: Choose exercises that you find enjoyable and engaging to increase the likelihood of sticking to your routine.

4. Create a schedule: Plan your workouts in advance

and make them a regular part of your daily routine.

5. Stay accountable: Enlist the support of friends or family members, join a workout group, or work with a personal trainer to stay accountable and motivated.

Recommended Exercises for Those with Limited Mobility

For individuals with limited mobility due to age or other causes, it's still possible to engage in physical activity. Here are some exercises that can be adapted to accommodate varying levels of mobility:

1. Seated exercises: Chair-based exercises, such as seated marches, seated leg lifts, or seated tap dance, can be performed to improve cardiovascular fitness, muscle strength, and flexibility.

2. Water-based exercises: Swimming, water aerobics, or water walking can provide low-impact exercise options that are gentle on joints and muscles.

3. Gentle stretching: Stretching exercises can be performed while sitting or lying down to maintain flexibility and joint mobility. Incorporate props such as straps, blocks, or pillows to support your body as needed.

4. Resistance band exercises: Resistance bands can be used for seated or lying-down exercises to strengthen various muscle groups while minimizing joint stress.

5. Tai chi or yoga: These mind-body practices can be adapted to meet individual needs, helping improve balance, flexibility, and strength while reducing stress and promoting relaxation.

Virtual Reality Exercise: A Fun and Engaging

Alternative

For those seeking a unique and engaging form of exercise, virtual reality (VR) fitness might be the perfect solution. Using a VR headset, such as the Meta Quest, allows you to immerse yourself in interactive games that get you moving and provide a fun workout experience.

One of the most popular VR games for exercise is Beat Saber. In this game, players wield virtual lightsabers to slash flying boxes in time with the music, all while dodging walls and obstacles. The result is a full-body workout that is both entertaining and challenging, making it an enjoyable way to incorporate physical activity into your daily routine.

Benefits of VR Exercise for Kidney Patients

Enjoyment: VR games, like Beat Saber, offer an entertaining alternative to traditional exercise, making it easier to stay motivated and maintain a consistent workout routine.

1. Low impact: Many VR games involve moderate-intensity movements that are low impact, making them suitable for individuals with kidney disease who may need to avoid high-intensity or high-impact exercises.

2. Customizable: VR games often come with adjustable settings, allowing you to tailor the intensity and difficulty of the game to suit your fitness level and preferences.

3. Accessibility: VR exercise can be done in the comfort of your own home, making it a convenient option for those with limited access to fitness facilities or outdoor spaces.

4. Social support: Some VR games offer multiplayer options, allowing you to connect with friends or other players online, providing a social element and

additional motivation.

Tips for Incorporating VR Exercise into Your Routine

Consult your healthcare team: Before starting any new exercise program, discuss your plans with your healthcare team to ensure it's appropriate for your current health and kidney function.

1. Start slowly: Begin with shorter sessions and gradually increase the duration and intensity of your VR workouts as your fitness level improves.//
2. Set realistic goals: Establish achievable goals for your VR exercise routine, such as playing for a specific amount of time or reaching a certain level in the game.
3. Mix it up: To maintain interest and prevent boredom, explore various VR games and activities to find the ones you enjoy most and that provide a well-rounded workout.
4. Listen to your body: Pay attention to how your body feels during and after VR exercise sessions. If you experience any discomfort, pain, or unusual symptoms, stop the activity and consult your healthcare team.

Exercise and physical activity are essential components of a kidney-friendly lifestyle, offering numerous benefits for individuals with CKD. By working with your healthcare team to develop a personalized exercise plan, you can enjoy the advantages of regular physical activity while managing your kidney disease effectively. Remember to start gradually, set realistic goals, and choose activities you enjoy to help make exercise an enjoyable and sustainable part of your life.

BAKING SODA AND CKD

When it comes to kidney disease, there is no shortage of myths and misconceptions surrounding potential treatments and remedies. One such topic that often sparks debate is the role of baking soda, or sodium bicarbonate, in managing kidney disease. This chapter will provide an in-depth exploration of baking soda and kidney disease, debunking myths, discussing its potential benefits and limitations, and examining the current research on this topic.

What is Baking Soda

Baking soda, also known as sodium bicarbonate, is a chemical compound commonly found in the form of a white, crystalline powder. It is an alkaline substance that can neutralize acids, making it a popular ingredient in many household and culinary applications, including baking, cleaning, and even as an antacid for heartburn relief.

However, beyond its everyday uses, baking soda has also been the subject of scientific research for its potential role in managing kidney disease. It is crucial to separate fact from fiction and understand the science behind baking soda's effects on kidney health.

Baking Soda and Kidney Disease: Separating Fact from Fiction

First and foremost, it is essential to debunk a widespread myth: baking soda is not a cure for kidney disease. Kidney disease is a complex condition with multiple contributing factors and various stages of progression. There is currently no cure for kidney disease, and any claims suggesting that baking soda can reverse or cure kidney damage are misleading and not supported by scientific evidence.

That being said, baking soda does have a specific role in managing kidney disease, particularly in cases where a patient's bicarbonate levels are low. To understand this role, it is necessary to delve into the science of kidney function and acid-base balance in the body.

The Role of Bicarbonate in Kidney Function

The kidneys play a vital role in maintaining the body's acid-base balance by filtering and excreting excess acids and reabsorbing bicarbonate, an alkaline substance, back into the bloodstream. This balance is essential for optimal cellular function and overall health. In healthy individuals, the kidneys work efficiently to maintain normal bicarbonate levels, which typically range between 22 and 29 milliequivalents per liter (mEq/L).

However, in individuals with kidney disease, the kidneys' ability to filter and reabsorb bicarbonate may become impaired, leading to a condition known as metabolic acidosis. Metabolic acidosis occurs when the body's bicarbonate levels drop below 22 mEq/L, causing an acidic environment in the body. This can result in various symptoms and complications, including rapid breathing, confusion, fatigue, and muscle weakness. Furthermore, chronic metabolic acidosis can exacerbate kidney damage and accelerate the progression of kidney disease.

The Role of Baking Soda in Managing Metabolic Acidosis

Given that baking soda is a source of bicarbonate, it has been investigated as a potential treatment for metabolic acidosis in individuals with kidney disease. The idea is that by supplementing with sodium bicarbonate, a patient's bicarbonate levels can be increased, neutralizing excess acids and helping to maintain a healthy acid-base balance in the body.

It is essential to note that baking soda supplementation is not appropriate for all individuals with kidney disease, nor is it a one-size-fits-all solution. The decision to use baking soda as part of a kidney disease treatment plan should be made on a case-by-case basis, taking into account the patient's specific needs, stage of kidney disease, and underlying health conditions.

Current Research on Baking Soda and Kidney Disease

Several studies have investigated the potential benefits of baking soda supplementation in individuals with kidney disease, particularly in those with low bicarbonate levels. While the research is still ongoing, some studies have shown promising results.

A study published in the Journal of the American Society of Nephrology in 2009 found that daily sodium bicarbonate supplementation in patients with metabolic acidosis and stage 4 chronic kidney disease (CKD) significantly slowed the decline of kidney function compared to a control group receiving standard care. Furthermore, the study reported that participants receiving sodium bicarbonate supplementation experienced a lower incidence of rapid kidney function decline and a reduced need for dialysis initiation.

Another study, published in 2015 in the Clinical Journal of the American Society of Nephrology, showed that sodium bicarbonate supplementation in patients with stage 3 CKD and low serum bicarbonate levels led to improvements in kidney function and slowed the progression of kidney disease.

While these findings are encouraging, it is important to note that not all studies have shown the same positive results, and **more research is needed** to fully understand the potential benefits and limitations of baking soda supplementation in kidney disease management.

Considerations and Precautions

As with any treatment or intervention, there are several factors to consider before incorporating baking soda into a kidney disease management plan:

1. Consult a healthcare professional: As previously mentioned, baking soda supplementation is not suitable for all individuals with kidney disease. It is crucial to consult with a nephrologist or renal dietitian before making any changes to your treatment plan.

2. Monitor sodium intake: Baking soda is a source of sodium, and individuals with kidney disease often need to limit their sodium intake to manage blood pressure and fluid balance. If baking soda supplementation is recommended, it is essential to account for the additional sodium in your overall diet and make adjustments as needed under the guidance of a renal dietitian.

3. Monitor potassium levels: In some cases, baking soda supplementation can cause a shift in the body's potassium levels. If you have kidney disease, it is crucial to closely monitor your potassium levels and make dietary adjustments as needed.

4. Start with a low dose: If your healthcare team recommends baking soda supplementation, it is typically advised to start with a low dose and gradually increase as needed, based on your bicarbonate levels and tolerance.

5. Adhere to the recommended dosing schedule: Baking soda supplementation should be taken as directed by your healthcare provider, typically in

divided doses throughout the day, to ensure optimal absorption and effectiveness.

While baking soda is not a cure for kidney disease, it does have a potential role in managing metabolic acidosis in individuals with low bicarbonate levels. However, this intervention should only be considered under the guidance of a healthcare professional, as part of a comprehensive and personalized treatment plan.

ANEMIA

Anemia is a common and often debilitating complication of chronic kidney disease (CKD). It can significantly impact a person's quality of life, making everyday activities challenging and reducing overall well-being. As a kidney patient, dealing with anemia was the most challenging symptom I faced. By working closely with my healthcare team and dietitian, I was able to address my iron deficiency and eventually eliminate my anemia. This chapter aims to provide a detailed overview of anemia in CKD, its causes, symptoms, management strategies, and tips for living with anemia.

Understanding Anemia in CKD

Anemia is a condition characterized by a shortage of red blood cells or a lack of hemoglobin, the protein in red blood cells responsible for carrying oxygen to the body's tissues. This shortage impairs the blood's ability to deliver adequate oxygen to the body, leading to fatigue, shortness of breath, and other symptoms.

In the context of CKD, anemia is primarily caused by a decrease in the production of erythropoietin (EPO), a hormone produced by the kidneys that stimulates the production of red blood cells in the bone marrow. As kidney function declines, EPO production decreases, leading to a reduction in red blood cell production and the development of anemia.

Other factors that can contribute to anemia in CKD include:

Iron deficiency: Iron is a critical component of hemoglobin, and insufficient iron intake or absorption can lead to anemia. CKD patients may have lower iron stores due to dietary restrictions, blood loss during hemodialysis, or inflammation that impairs iron absorption.

Vitamin deficiencies: Adequate levels of vitamin B12 and folic acid are necessary for red blood cell production. Deficiencies in these vitamins, which may result from dietary restrictions or poor absorption, can contribute to anemia in CKD patients.

Inflammation: Chronic inflammation, common in CKD, can suppress red blood cell production and shorten the lifespan of existing red blood cells.

Blood loss: Hemodialysis can lead to minor blood loss, which, over time, can contribute to anemia.

Symptoms of Anemia in CKD

Anemia can cause a range of symptoms that impact daily functioning and quality of life, including:

- Fatigue and weakness
- Shortness of breath
- Dizziness and lightheadedness
- Difficulty concentrating and reduced cognitive function
- Pale skin
- Chest pain and rapid heartbeat, particularly during physical activity
- Cold hands and feet
- Headaches
- Insomnia or difficulty sleeping

Management Strategies for Anemia in CKD

Effectively managing anemia in CKD requires a multifaceted approach, which may include:

Iron supplementation: Oral or intravenous iron supplements can help address iron deficiency and improve anemia symptoms. A dietitian can help determine the appropriate form and dosage of iron supplementation, depending on individual needs and circumstances. Switching to cast iron cookware can also increase the iron in your diet.

Erythropoiesis-stimulating agents (ESAs): ESAs are medications that mimic the effects of EPO, stimulating red blood cell production. These medications can be prescribed by a healthcare provider to help manage anemia in CKD patients, particularly those undergoing dialysis.

Blood transfusions: In severe cases of anemia, blood transfusions may be necessary to increase red blood cell levels quickly.

Vitamin supplementation: If vitamin B12 or folic acid deficiency is contributing to anemia, supplementation with these vitamins may be recommended.

Dietary modifications: A renal dietitian can help create a balanced, kidney-friendly diet plan that provides adequate iron, vitamin B12, and folic acid while considering other dietary restrictions necessary for CKD management.

Addressing inflammation: Identifying and addressing the causes of inflammation in CKD patients, such as infections or autoimmune disorders, can help improve anemia management.

Monitoring and adjusting medications: Some medications prescribed for CKD patients, such as phosphate binders, can interfere with iron absorption. Regular monitoring and adjustments to medications may be necessary to optimize anemia management.

Tips for Living with Anemia in CKD

Managing anemia in CKD can be challenging, but by working closely with a healthcare team and dietitian, it is possible to improve symptoms and quality of life. Here are some tips for living with anemia in CKD:

Communicate with your healthcare team: Keep your healthcare team informed about your symptoms and any changes in your condition. Regular check-ups and lab tests can help your team make necessary adjustments to your treatment plan.

Follow dietary recommendations: Work with a renal dietitian to ensure you are consuming an appropriate diet that provides necessary nutrients for managing anemia while still being kidney-friendly.

Prioritize rest and self-care: Anemia can cause significant fatigue, making it important to prioritize rest and self-care. Listen to your body and allow yourself time to rest when needed.

Engage in gentle exercise: Engaging in gentle, low-impact exercise, such as walking or yoga, can help improve energy levels and overall well-being. Consult with your healthcare team before starting a new exercise routine.

Manage stress: Chronic stress can exacerbate anemia symptoms, making it essential to incorporate stress management techniques into your daily routine. Meditation, deep breathing exercises, and mindfulness practices can help reduce stress and promote relaxation.

Stay informed: Educate yourself about anemia and CKD to better understand your condition and the steps you can take to manage it effectively. Stay up to date on the latest research and advancements in CKD and anemia treatment.

Seek support: Living with anemia and CKD can be challenging, but you don't have to face it alone. Reach out to friends, family members, or support groups to share your experiences, seek advice, and find encouragement.

BUBBLES IN YOUR URINE

The appearance of bubbles in urine can be a perplexing and somewhat disconcerting sight. For some, it may even raise concerns about kidney health. In this chapter, we will delve into the fascinating world of urine bubbles, exploring common causes and why it's rarely a sign of kidney issues. Rest assured, by the end of this chapter, you'll have a clear understanding of bubbles in urine and how to approach this bubbly phenomenon.

Common Causes of Bubbles in Urine

1. Speedy stream: One of the most common explanations for bubbles in urine is the force with which the urine is expelled. A strong, high-velocity stream can create air bubbles as it hits the water in the toilet. In this case, the bubbles are harmless and unrelated to any health issue.

2. Dehydration: Dehydration can cause your urine to become more concentrated, which increases the likelihood of bubbles forming. When you're dehydrated, your body retains more water, resulting in less fluid in your urine. This can also cause your urine to be darker in color and have a stronger odor. Ensuring proper hydration can help alleviate this issue.

3. Proteinuria: Although it's not the most common cause, bubbles in urine can be due to excess

protein (proteinuria). In healthy individuals, the kidneys filter out waste products while keeping essential proteins in the bloodstream. However, if the kidneys are not functioning optimally, they may allow protein to leak into the urine, creating bubbles. Proteinuria is a possible symptom of kidney disease, but it is important to note that bubbles in the urine alone are not a definitive sign of kidney issues.

4. Presence of soap: Bubbles in urine can sometimes be attributed to residual soap or cleaning products in the toilet bowl. When urine mixes with these substances, it can create bubbles that give the appearance of foamy urine. This cause is entirely harmless and unrelated to your health.

5. Medications: Some medications can cause urine to become frothy or bubbly. Diuretics, for example, increase the volume of urine and can create bubbles as a side effect. If you suspect your medication is causing bubbles in your urine, consult with your healthcare provider for advice.

6. Urinary Tract Infections (UTIs): Occur when pesky bacteria enter the urinary system, causing inflammation—usually in the bladder or urethra. These infections can give rise to various symptoms, such as painful or frequent urination, cloudy or strong-smelling urine, and the enigmatic presence of bubbles in the urine. These bubbles can result from gas release by bacteria in the urinary tract or from the interaction between urine and mucus produced by the inflamed urinary tract. To treat UTIs, a course of antibiotics prescribed by a healthcare professional typically does the trick.

7. Retrograde Ejaculation: In men, retrograde

ejaculation is a peculiar phenomenon that occurs when semen enters the bladder rather than being expelled through the urethra during ejaculation. This condition can cause semen to mingle with urine, leading to the appearance of bubbles when urinating. Retrograde ejaculation can stem from various causes, including nerve damage, prostate surgery, or the use of certain medications. Although generally not harmful, this condition can cause fertility issues for men trying to conceive.

8. Vesicocolic Fistula: An abnormal and infrequent connection between the colon and the bladder. This rare condition can cause gas from the colon to enter the bladder, leading to the presence of bubbles in the urine. Other symptoms of a vesicocolic fistula may include recurrent UTIs, abdominal pain, and fecal material in the urine. Treatment for a vesicocolic fistula typically involves surgical repair to close the connection between the colon and the bladder.

Bubbles in Urine: Rarely a Sign of Kidney Issues

While bubbles in the urine can be attributed to various causes, it is important to emphasize that their presence rarely indicates kidney issues. If you have concerns about your kidney health, it is essential to consult your healthcare team and undergo the appropriate tests. Relying solely on the presence of bubbles in your urine as an indicator of kidney health is not an accurate or reliable method.

If you have concerns about your kidney health, don't hesitate to reach out to your healthcare team. They can provide guidance, perform appropriate tests, and ensure you receive the care you need. In the meantime, you can continue to marvel at the mysterious and captivating world of urine bubbles.

GOUT AND URIC ACID

Gout is an excruciating and incapacitating type of inflammatory arthritis that plagues millions of individuals worldwide. The root of this agony lies in the buildup of uric acid in the blood, which subsequently forms urate crystals in the joints and surrounding tissues. This chapter delves into the intricate relationship between gout and uric acid, exploring the causes, risk factors, symptoms, and available treatments. Our goal is to provide you with valuable insights to better comprehend and manage this condition effectively.

The Uric Acid Saga

Uric acid is a waste byproduct stemming from the breakdown of purines, organic compounds present in certain foods, beverages, and our body's cells. The kidneys play a pivotal role in filtering uric acid from the blood and expelling it through urine. However, when the body generates excessive uric acid or the kidneys struggle to remove it efficiently, hyperuricemia—elevated uric acid levels in the blood—occurs.

Hyperuricemia and the Emergence of Gout

Hyperuricemia is a primary risk factor for gout development. As uric acid levels in the blood rise, urate crystals form in joints, tendons, and surrounding tissues, inducing inflammation and pain—gout's signature symptoms.

The Culprits: Causes and Risk Factors for Gout

Several elements can contribute to gout development and increased uric acid levels:

- Genetics: A family history of gout elevates your risk.
- Age and gender: Gout predominantly affects men and becomes more prevalent with age.
- Diet: Consuming purine-rich foods, such as red meat, organ meats, seafood, and alcohol, can raise uric acid levels.
- Obesity: Excess weight can lead to increased uric acid production and decreased kidney efficiency.
- Medications: Diuretics and low-dose aspirin, among others, can heighten uric acid levels.
- Medical conditions: Kidney disease, diabetes, hypertension, and metabolic syndrome increase gout risk.
- Surgery or trauma: Gout can occasionally be triggered by surgery or severe injury.

Symptoms of Gout: An Unwanted Visitor

Gout attacks often strike suddenly, characterized by intense pain, swelling, redness, and warmth in the affected joint. Although the big toe is a frequent target, gout can also impact the ankle, knee, wrist, and elbow. Gout attacks typically occur at night and persist for several days.

Between gout attacks, individuals might not experience any symptoms. However, without proper management, gout can progress, leading to joint damage and chronic pain.

Diagnosing Gout: The Investigation

To diagnose gout, healthcare providers gather a detailed medical history, perform a physical examination, and may order laboratory tests to assess uric acid levels in the blood and joint fluid analysis to confirm urate crystal presence.

Imaging studies, such as X-rays, ultrasound, or dual-energy computed tomography (DECT), can be instrumental in detecting joint damage and identifying urate crystals.

Gout Treatment: Alleviating Pain and Preventing Flare-Ups

Gout treatment aims to mitigate pain during acute attacks, avert future attacks, and minimize complications. Treatment options include:

1. Medications: NSAIDs, corticosteroids, and colchicine are commonly utilized to relieve pain and inflammation during acute gout attacks.

2. Urate-lowering therapy: Allopurinol, febuxostat, and probenecid help reduce uric acid production or increase excretion, preventing future gout attacks and complications.

3. Lifestyle changes: Diet modifications, weight management, hydration, and alcohol consumption limits can reduce uric acid levels and gout attack risk.

4. Managing comorbidities: Controlling conditions such as diabetes, high blood pressure, and kidney disease can help reduce gout risk and complications.

Dietary Recommendations for Gout Management

Adopting dietary changes can aid in lowering uric acid levels and reducing the risk of gout attacks. Here are some general dietary guidelines for individuals with gout:

1. Limit high-purine foods: Purine-rich foods like red meat, organ meats, and certain types of seafood can increase uric acid levels. Opt for lean protein sources like poultry, fish, and plant-based proteins instead.

2. Avoid sugary beverages and foods: High-fructose

corn syrup, found in numerous processed foods and beverages, has been linked to an increased risk of gout. Choose water, herbal tea, or low-sugar beverages, and consume whole, unprocessed foods when possible.

3. Limit alcohol intake: Alcohol, particularly beer, can contribute to elevated uric acid levels. If you decide to drink, opt for moderate consumption of wine or spirits and avoid binge drinking.
4. Increase intake of low-purine vegetables: Vegetables are low in purines and provide essential nutrients for overall health. Incorporate a variety of colorful vegetables into your diet, such as leafy greens, bell peppers, tomatoes, and carrots.
5. Consume low-fat dairy products: Research indicates that low-fat dairy products can help reduce the risk of gout. Include low-fat milk, yogurt, and cheese in your diet.
6. Stay hydrated: Drinking sufficient water helps flush excess uric acid from the body, decreasing the risk of crystal formation.
7. Choose whole grains: Whole grains like brown rice, quinoa, and whole wheat are healthier choices than refined grains and can promote overall health.

Understanding the relationship between gout and uric acid is crucial for effectively managing this condition. By following the guidelines outlined in this chapter, you can take proactive steps to reduce the risk of gout attacks and improve your overall well-being.

KIDNEY STONES

Kidney stones, or renal calculi, are hard deposits comprised of minerals and salts that form within the kidneys. These stones can differ in size and shape and may cause immense pain when passing through the urinary tract. While kidney stones are a common occurrence, they can lead to complications, particularly for those with kidney disease. This chapter aims to provide an in-depth understanding of kidney stones, their formation, causes, symptoms, treatment options, and prevention strategies.

Formation and Types of Kidney Stones

Kidney stones form when urine becomes concentrated, allowing minerals and salts to crystallize and bind together. There are four primary types of kidney stones:

1. Calcium stones: These are the most prevalent type of kidney stones, accounting for approximately 80% of cases. Calcium stones are typically composed of calcium oxalate, although calcium phosphate stones also exist.

2. Uric acid stones: These stones develop when there is a high concentration of uric acid in the urine. Uric acid stones are more prevalent in men and may be associated with gout, a type of arthritis caused by an excess of uric acid in the bloodstream.

3. Struvite stones: Struvite stones result from urinary tract infections and are more common in women. These stones can grow considerably large and cause

significant pain.

4. Cystine stones: Cystine stones are rare and occur in individuals with a genetic disorder called cystinuria. This disorder causes the kidneys to excrete excessive amounts of the amino acid cystine, leading to stone formation.

Causes and Risk Factors

Several factors can contribute to the formation of kidney stones, including:

Dehydration: Insufficient water intake can lead to concentrated urine, increasing the risk of kidney stone formation.

Diet: A diet high in protein, sodium, and oxalate-rich foods can contribute to the formation of kidney stones.

Obesity: Excess body weight is associated with a higher risk of developing kidney stones.

Family history: A family history of kidney stones may increase your likelihood of developing them.

Medical conditions: Certain medical conditions, such as inflammatory bowel disease, hyperparathyroidism, and renal tubular acidosis, can increase the risk of kidney stones.

Symptoms

Kidney stones often cause no symptoms when they remain in the kidney. However, when a stone moves into the ureter (the tube connecting the kidney and bladder), symptoms may include:

- Severe pain in the back, abdomen, or side
- Blood in the urine
- Nausea and vomiting
- Frequent urination
- Painful urination

- Cloudy or foul-smelling urine

If you suspect you have a kidney stone, it is crucial to seek medical attention. A healthcare professional will diagnose kidney stones through a physical examination, urine tests, blood tests, and imaging studies such as X-rays or CT scans.

Treatment

Treatment for kidney stones depends on the size and location of the stone, as well as the severity of symptoms. Some common treatment options include:

1. Pain management: Over-the-counter pain relievers or prescription medications may be used to alleviate pain.
2. Fluid intake: Drinking plenty of water can help flush out smaller stones.
3. Medical therapy: Certain medications can help break down and pass kidney stones.
4. Extracorporeal shock wave lithotripsy (ESWL): This non-invasive procedure uses sound waves to break up large stones, allowing them to pass more easily.
5. Ureteroscopy: A thin tube is inserted into the ureter to remove or break up the stone.
6. Percutaneous nephrolithotomy: In this surgical procedure, a small incision is made in the back to remove large kidney stones directly from the kidney.
7. Parathyroid surgery: If a stone is caused by hyperparathyroidism, surgery to remove the overactive parathyroid gland may be necessary.

Prevention Strategies

Preventing kidney stones involves making lifestyle and dietary changes to reduce the risk factors associated with stone formation. Here are some tips to help prevent kidney stones:

Stay hydrated: Aim to drink at least 8 to 10 cups of water per day. Staying well-hydrated helps dilute the substances in urine that can lead to kidney stones.

Limit sodium intake: Consuming high levels of sodium can increase the risk of kidney stones. Aim for a daily sodium intake of less than 2,300 mg, or even lower if you have a history of kidney stones.

Moderate protein consumption: A high-protein diet can increase the risk of kidney stones, especially uric acid stones. Consider limiting animal protein sources and incorporating plant-based proteins instead.

Consume calcium-rich foods: Adequate calcium intake from food sources may help reduce the risk of calcium oxalate stones. However, be cautious with calcium supplements, as excessive supplementation can increase the risk of stone formation.

Limit oxalate-rich foods: Foods high in oxalates, such as spinach, rhubarb, beets, and nuts, can contribute to calcium oxalate stones. Limiting these foods and consuming them with calcium-rich foods can help reduce the risk.

Maintain a healthy body weight: Obesity is a risk factor for kidney stones. Adopting a balanced diet and engaging in regular physical activity can help maintain a healthy weight.

Manage medical conditions: If you have a medical condition that increases your risk of kidney stones, work with your healthcare provider to manage the condition effectively. Proper management of underlying medical issues can help reduce the risk of kidney stones and associated complications.

Understanding the formation, causes, symptoms, and treatment options for kidney stones can help individuals better manage and prevent this painful condition. Making lifestyle and dietary changes, staying hydrated, and addressing underlying medical conditions are crucial strategies for reducing the risk of kidney stones and maintaining overall kidney health.

ITCHY SKIN AND CKD

Itchy skin, also known as pruritus, is a common and frustrating symptom experienced by many people with chronic kidney disease (CKD). While high phosphorus levels can contribute to itchy skin, it's essential to recognize that there are numerous other possible causes. This chapter will explore the various factors that may lead to itchy skin in CKD patients and provide practical tips for addressing and alleviating this troublesome symptom.

Possible Causes of Itchy Skin in CKD Patients

High Phosphorus Levels: As kidney function declines, the ability to remove excess phosphorus from the body decreases, leading to high phosphorus levels in the blood. This can cause itching, particularly in patients with severely reduced kidney function.

Dry Skin: CKD patients often experience dry skin due to a decrease in sweat and oil gland function. Dry skin can be itchy and uncomfortable.

Uremic Pruritus: Uremic pruritus is a type of itching caused by the accumulation of waste products in the body due to decreased kidney function. This type of itching can be severe and widespread.

Allergies: Allergies to certain medications, soaps, or skincare products can cause itching and skin irritation in some individuals.

Liver Disease: Liver disease can also cause itching, as the liver plays a role in processing toxins and waste products.

High Phosphorus Levels

High phosphorus levels can cause itchy skin in CKD patients due to a condition known as hyperphosphatemia. When the kidneys are functioning properly, they efficiently remove excess phosphorus from the body. However, in CKD patients, the kidneys' ability to filter out and maintain the right balance of phosphorus is impaired, leading to a buildup of phosphorus in the blood.

When phosphorus levels in the blood become too high, the body tries to maintain a balance by pulling calcium from the bones. As a result, the calcium and phosphorus in the blood can bind together, forming calcium-phosphate crystals. These crystals can deposit in the skin and other soft tissues, causing inflammation and irritation that leads to itching.

Furthermore, the excess phosphorus in the bloodstream can also contribute to the development of secondary hyperparathyroidism. In response to the imbalance of calcium and phosphorus, the parathyroid glands release more parathyroid hormone (PTH), which can exacerbate the itching sensation.

Tips for Addressing Itchy Skin

Moisturize Regularly: Apply a gentle, fragrance-free moisturizer to your skin at least twice a day, especially after bathing. This will help combat dry skin and reduce itching.

Avoid Hot Showers: Hot water can strip the skin of its natural oils, making it more prone to dryness and itching. Opt for lukewarm water instead and keep showers short.

Use Mild Soaps: Choose mild, fragrance-free soaps and laundry detergents to minimize skin irritation.

Avoid Scratching: Scratching can damage the skin and worsen itching. Try to resist the urge to scratch, and consider using a cold or damp cloth to soothe the affected area instead.

Stay Hydrated: Drinking plenty of water can help improve skin hydration and may reduce itching.

Manage Phosphorus Levels: Work with your healthcare team and dietitian to monitor and manage your phosphorus levels through diet and medications, if needed.

Address Underlying Causes: If you suspect allergies or another underlying cause for your itchy skin, consult with your healthcare team to identify and address the issue.

Over-the-Counter Remedies: In some cases, over-the-counter creams containing hydrocortisone or antihistamines may help alleviate itching. Always consult your healthcare team before using any new medications or treatments.

SLEEPLESS NIGHTS AND KIDNEY HEALTH

A good night's sleep is essential for maintaining overall health and well-being. Unfortunately, many people with chronic kidney disease (CKD) experience sleep disturbances, which can negatively impact their quality of life. This chapter will explore the common causes of sleep issues in CKD patients, offer solutions to address them, provide tips for better sleep, and discuss the potential benefits of using melatonin.

Causes of Sleep Issues in CKD Patients

There are several factors that contribute to sleep disturbances in individuals with CKD:

Sleep Apnea: Sleep apnea is a common condition among CKD patients. It is characterized by frequent pauses in breathing during sleep, leading to poor sleep quality.

Restless Legs Syndrome (RLS): RLS is a neurological disorder that causes an irresistible urge to move the legs, often accompanied by uncomfortable sensations. It can disrupt sleep and is more common in people with CKD.

Insomnia: Difficulty falling or staying asleep, known as insomnia, is prevalent among CKD patients, often due to pain, anxiety, or depression.

Chronic Pain: Pain associated with kidney disease or other underlying health conditions can make it difficult for CKD patients to fall asleep or stay asleep.

Solutions to Address Sleep Issues

Addressing the underlying causes of sleep disturbances can significantly improve sleep quality in CKD patients:

Sleep Apnea: Consult a healthcare professional to diagnose and treat sleep apnea. Continuous positive airway pressure (CPAP) therapy is the most common treatment, which involves wearing a mask that delivers air pressure to keep the airways open during sleep.

Restless Legs Syndrome: Treatments for RLS include iron supplementation, medication adjustments, and adopting a healthy lifestyle that includes regular exercise and relaxation techniques.

Insomnia: Cognitive-behavioral therapy, relaxation techniques, and creating a sleep-friendly environment can help alleviate insomnia. Discuss any medications that may contribute to insomnia with your healthcare provider.

Chronic Pain: Work with your healthcare team to develop a pain management plan, which may include medications, physical therapy, or alternative treatments like acupuncture.

Tips for Better Sleep

1. Maintain a consistent sleep schedule by going to bed and waking up at the same time every day.
2. Create a comfortable and relaxing sleep environment, free from noise, bright lights, and extreme temperatures.
3. Limit exposure to screens (TV, computer, smartphone) at least one hour before bedtime.
4. Engage in relaxing activities before bed, such as reading, listening to calming music, or taking a warm bath.
5. Avoid caffeine and alcohol close to bedtime, as they

can disrupt sleep.

6. Exercise regularly, but avoid vigorous exercise close to bedtime, as it may stimulate the body and make it more difficult to fall asleep.
7. Limit daytime naps, as they can interfere with nighttime sleep. If you must nap, keep it short (20-30 minutes) and in the early afternoon.
8. Avoid large meals and spicy foods close to bedtime, as they can cause indigestion and disrupt sleep.
9. Use relaxation techniques, such as deep breathing exercises, progressive muscle relaxation, or meditation, to help calm the mind and prepare the body for sleep.
10. Consider seeking professional help if your sleep issues persist, as they may be indicative of an underlying health condition or require specialized treatment.

Melatonin and CKD

Melatonin is a hormone that regulates sleep-wake cycles. Research suggests that melatonin supplementation may improve sleep quality in CKD patients. A study by Koch et al. (2009) found that melatonin supplementation significantly reduced sleep latency (time taken to fall asleep) and increased total sleep time in CKD patients with insomnia. However, further research is needed to confirm these findings and determine the optimal dosage and duration of melatonin supplementation for CKD patients.

It is essential to discuss the use of melatonin with your healthcare provider before starting supplementation, as it may interact with certain medications or cause side effects in some individuals.

The Importance of Addressing Sleep Issues in

CKD Patients

In addition to negatively impacting overall quality of life, sleep disturbances in CKD patients can lead to more severe health problems. Poor sleep has been linked to an increased risk of cardiovascular events, worsening kidney function, and a higher mortality rate among CKD patients (Roumelioti et al., 2011). Therefore, it is crucial to take sleep issues seriously and work with your healthcare team to develop a comprehensive plan for improving your sleep quality.

References:

Roumelioti, M. E., Buysse, D. J., Sanders, M. H., Strollo, P., Newman, A. B., & Unruh, M. L. (2011). Sleep-disordered breathing and excessive daytime sleepiness in chronic kidney disease and hemodialysis. Clinical Journal of the American Society of Nephrology, 6(5), 986-994. https://doi.org/10.2215/CJN.08110910

UNDERSTANDING KIDNEY PAIN

It's not uncommon for people to confuse kidney pain with back pain, which can lead to unnecessary worry and confusion. In this chapter, we'll delve into the distinctions between kidney pain and back pain, explore the possible causes of kidney pain, and discuss when to seek medical attention. Recognizing the differences between these types of pain is crucial for making informed decisions about your health and ensuring proper diagnosis and treatment.

Distinguishing Kidney Pain from Back Pain

To differentiate kidney pain from back pain, it's essential to understand the kidneys' location. These two bean-shaped organs are situated in the lower back, just below the ribcage, on either side of the spine. Kidney pain, also referred to as renal pain, generally occurs in the area where the kidneys are located.

Back pain, conversely, can arise from various causes, such as muscle strain, ligament sprains, spinal disc problems, or even poor posture. It typically occurs in the middle or lower back and can be felt on one or both sides of the spine.

Characteristics of Kidney Pain

Kidney pain often presents as a dull, constant ache, or a sharp, severe, and sudden pain. It usually occurs on one side of the lower back, beneath the ribs, and may radiate to the groin or abdominal area. Other symptoms that may accompany kidney pain include fever, nausea, vomiting, and changes in urinary habits (such as increased frequency or a decrease in the amount of urine).

Characteristics of Back Pain

Back pain can vary in intensity, ranging from a mild, dull ache to a sharp, stabbing sensation. It typically occurs in the lower or middle back but may also be felt in the upper back or neck. Back pain may be accompanied by muscle stiffness, limited range of motion, or radiating pain down the legs. In some cases, back pain may be worsened by specific movements or positions.

Potential Causes of Kidney Pain

Kidney stones: These small, hard deposits of minerals and salts form in the kidneys and can cause severe pain when passing through the urinary tract.

Kidney infection (pyelonephritis): Bacterial infections in one or both kidneys can cause pain, fever, chills, and frequent, painful urination.

Polycystic kidney disease (PKD): This genetic disorder leads to the development of fluid-filled cysts in the kidneys, causing kidney pain, high blood pressure, and kidney failure.

Kidney trauma: An injury to the kidneys can result from a direct blow to the back, a fall, or a car accident, leading to pain and potential kidney damage.

Kidney cancer: While kidney cancer is often asymptomatic in its early stages, it may cause pain in the back or side as the tumor grows.

Glomerulonephritis: Inflammation of the kidney's filtering units (glomeruli) can cause pain, accompanied by symptoms like swelling, high blood pressure, and changes in urine color.

Renal artery stenosis: The narrowing of the renal artery, which supplies blood to the kidneys, can cause kidney pain, high blood pressure, and decreased kidney function.

Common Causes of Back Pain

Muscle or ligament strain: Overexertion, improper lifting, or sudden movements can strain the muscles and ligaments in the back, leading to pain.

Disc problems: Spinal discs, which serve as cushions between the vertebrae, can bulge or rupture, causing pain, inflammation, and sometimes nerve irritation.

Arthritis: Osteoarthritis, the most common form of arthritis, can cause pain and stiffness in the joints of the spine.

Osteoporosis: This bone-weakening disease can lead to compression fractures in the spine, resulting in back pain.

Poor posture: Prolonged periods of sitting or standing with poor posture can strain the muscles, ligaments, and discs in the back, leading to pain.

Scoliosis: An abnormal curvature of the spine can cause muscle imbalances and pain in the back.

Sciatica: Irritation or compression of the sciatic nerve can cause pain that radiates from the lower back down the leg.

Spinal stenosis: Narrowing of the spinal canal can put pressure on the spinal cord and nerves, causing pain, numbness, and weakness in the back and legs.

Spondylolisthesis: This condition occurs when a vertebra slips out of place and puts pressure on the spinal nerves, resulting in pain.

When to Seek Medical Attention for Kidney Pain or Back Pain

If you experience persistent or severe pain in your back or sides, it's essential to consult with a healthcare professional. The following situations warrant immediate medical attention:

- Severe, sudden pain that does not improve with rest

or over-the-counter pain relievers.
- Pain accompanied by fever, chills, nausea, vomiting, or changes in urinary habits.
- Pain that radiates down the legs or causes numbness, tingling, or weakness in the legs.
- Pain following a fall, accident, or injury.
- Pain that interferes with daily activities or sleep.

By understanding the differences between kidney pain and back pain, as well as their potential causes, you can make more informed decisions about your health and ensure proper diagnosis and treatment. If you are concerned about pain in your back or sides, don't hesitate to reach out to a healthcare professional for guidance and support.

LIFE EXPECTANCY OF THOSE WITH CKD

Living with kidney disease can be challenging, and one of the most common concerns among patients is the potential impact on life expectancy. While it is impossible to predict an individual's exact life expectancy, it is essential to understand that being proactive in maintaining a heart-healthy lifestyle and working closely with your healthcare team can significantly influence your quality of life and life expectancy.

Factors that Influence Life Expectancy

Several factors can impact the life expectancy of those with kidney disease, and understanding these factors can help you make informed decisions about your health and treatment plan.

Stage of kidney disease: The stage of kidney disease is a crucial factor in determining life expectancy. Earlier stages of kidney disease (stages 1 and 2) typically have a better prognosis than later stages (stages 4 and 5). Early diagnosis and intervention can help slow the progression of kidney disease and improve overall outcomes.

Age: Older individuals with kidney disease may experience a faster decline in kidney function, which can affect life expectancy. However, maintaining a healthy lifestyle and adhering to a kidney-friendly diet can help improve overall health and slow the progression of kidney disease, even in older patients.

Comorbidities: The presence of other chronic conditions, such as diabetes, hypertension, and cardiovascular disease, can impact life expectancy in individuals with kidney disease. Proper management of these conditions, in conjunction with a kidney-friendly diet and lifestyle, can help improve overall outcomes.

Lifestyle habits: Maintaining a heart-healthy lifestyle is critical for individuals with kidney disease. This includes following a balanced, kidney-friendly diet, engaging in regular physical activity, maintaining a healthy weight, managing stress, and avoiding harmful habits such as smoking and excessive alcohol consumption. Adopting these habits can help slow the progression of kidney disease and improve life expectancy.

Treatment adherence: Following your healthcare team's recommendations, including taking prescribed medications and adhering to dietary restrictions, plays a significant role in determining life expectancy. Staying proactive in your treatment plan and working closely with your healthcare team can help ensure the best possible outcomes.

Support system: A strong support system, including family, friends, and healthcare professionals, can have a positive impact on life expectancy. Emotional support and encouragement can help individuals with kidney disease stay motivated to follow their treatment plan and make healthy choices.

Improving Life Expectancy: What You Can Do

While it is impossible to predict an exact life expectancy, there are steps you can take to improve your overall health and outcomes when living with kidney disease:

Be proactive in your care: Stay informed about your kidney health, adhere to your treatment plan, and regularly communicate with your healthcare team. This proactive approach can help you make timely adjustments to your treatment plan and slow the progression of kidney disease.

Maintain a heart-healthy lifestyle: Focus on a balanced, kidney-friendly diet, regular physical activity, stress management, and avoiding harmful habits. These lifestyle changes can help improve your overall health and slow the progression of kidney disease.

Manage comorbidities: Work with your healthcare team to manage any existing chronic conditions, such as diabetes, hypertension, and cardiovascular disease. Proper management of these conditions can help improve overall health and life expectancy.

Seek support: Lean on your support system, including family, friends, and healthcare professionals, for encouragement and guidance. A strong support system can help you stay motivated and navigate the challenges of living with kidney disease.

Regular check-ups and monitoring: Stay vigilant about scheduling regular check-ups with your healthcare team to monitor your kidney function and overall health. Early detection of any changes in your kidney health can help you make timely adjustments to your treatment plan, ultimately improving your life expectancy.

Educate yourself: Be informed about kidney disease and available treatment options. Educating yourself about your condition can help you make more informed decisions about your care and better communicate with your healthcare team.

Advocate for yourself: Speak up about your concerns and needs when discussing your treatment plan with your healthcare team. By actively participating in your care, you can ensure that your treatment plan is tailored to your unique circumstances, ultimately improving your overall health and life expectancy.

Stay updated on advancements: Research on kidney disease is constantly evolving, with new treatment options and advancements being developed. Stay informed about the latest findings and discuss any relevant advancements with your healthcare team to ensure that your treatment plan remains up-to-date and effective.

Develop coping strategies: Living with kidney disease can be emotionally challenging, and it is essential to develop healthy coping strategies to manage stress and maintain a positive outlook. Engaging in activities such as meditation, journaling, or support groups can help you navigate the emotional aspects of living with kidney disease.

Focus on mental health: Your mental health is just as important as your physical health when it comes to managing kidney disease. Reach out to mental health professionals or support groups if you need help coping with the emotional aspects of your condition. Maintaining a positive mental state can help you stay motivated and committed to your treatment plan.

Set realistic goals: Establish achievable, realistic goals for yourself when it comes to managing your kidney disease. Breaking down your treatment plan into smaller, manageable steps can help you stay focused and motivated to make progress.

Celebrate your successes: Acknowledge and celebrate the milestones you achieve while managing your kidney disease, no matter how small. Celebrating your successes can help you maintain a positive mindset and motivate you to continue making healthy choices.

While there is no way to predict the exact life expectancy of someone with kidney disease, being proactive and taking control of your health can significantly impact your overall well-being and life expectancy. By focusing on maintaining a heart-healthy lifestyle, managing comorbidities, working closely with your healthcare team, and staying optimistic, you can positively influence your kidney health and live a fulfilling life despite your diagnosis.

AVOIDING KIDNEY MYTHS AND SCAMS

The Kidney Health Maze: Fact vs. Fiction

When you're first diagnosed with kidney disease, it can feel like you've entered a confusing labyrinth of information. On one hand, you have science-based kidney advice, and on the other, you're bombarded with false claims, scams, and outright dangerous recommendations. How can you tell the difference and avoid getting trapped in the maze of misinformation?

Beware of False Cures, Unproven Supplements, and One-Size-Fits-All Treatment Plans

One of the biggest pitfalls kidney patients may encounter is the allure of fake cures, unproven supplements, and one-size-fits-all treatment plans. Sadly, there's no magic potion or pill that will cure kidney disease, and any claims to the contrary are deceptive and potentially harmful. Each person's kidney journey is unique, and the key to managing kidney disease lies in working closely with a healthcare team to create a personalized treatment plan.

Myth-Busting: Setting the Record Straight

Let's shatter some common kidney myths and make sure we're on solid ground when it comes to kidney health:

Myth: Drinking more water can heal kidney disease.

Reality: While staying hydrated is essential for overall health, guzzling gallons of water won't cure kidney disease. In fact, overloading on fluids can put added strain on the kidneys and lead to complications. It's essential to follow your healthcare team's recommendations for fluid intake based on your specific needs.

Myth: Cranberry juice helps flush the kidneys.

Reality: Cranberries and their juice have long been touted for their urinary tract benefits, but there's no evidence to support the idea that they can cleanse or flush the kidneys. Plus, cranberry juice can be high in sugar and oxalates, which can contribute to kidney stones in some people. Stick with a balanced, kidney-friendly diet and follow your healthcare team's guidance.

Myth: Everyone with kidney disease must avoid potassium-rich foods.

Reality: Potassium is an essential nutrient, but its levels need to be carefully managed for people with kidney disease. However, not everyone with kidney disease has the same potassium requirements. Work with a renal dietitian to determine your individual potassium needs and create a tailored meal plan.

Myth: Certain foods or supplements heal kidneys.

Reality: While a healthy, balanced diet and proper supplementation can help support kidney function, there is no specific food or supplement that can "heal" damaged kidneys. It's essential to work closely with your healthcare team and follow a personalized nutrition plan tailored to your specific needs to optimize kidney health.

Myth: Kidney patients cannot use oil in their meals.

Reality: Kidney patients can use oil in their meals, but it is crucial to choose the right type of oil and consume it in moderation. Healthy oils, such as olive oil or avocado oil, can be part of a kidney-friendly diet, as they are high in heart-healthy monounsaturated fats. However, it's essential to monitor your overall fat intake and avoid unhealthy oils, like hydrogenated or trans fats, that can contribute to inflammation and heart disease.

Myth: The only treatment for kidney disease is dialysis.

Reality: Dialysis is not the only treatment option for kidney disease. Depending on the stage of kidney disease, severity, and other factors, various treatment options are available. These can include lifestyle changes, medication management, and, in some cases, kidney transplantation. Conservative management is another option, focusing on symptom management and maintaining the quality of life without undergoing dialysis or transplantation. It's essential to work with your healthcare team to determine the best treatment plan for your unique situation.

Navigating Kidney Myths and Scams with Confidence

As a kidney health coach, empowering kidney patients with accurate, science-based information is a top priority. Here are some tips to help you navigate the kidney health maze and avoid scams:

Consult your healthcare team: Before making any significant changes to your diet, lifestyle, or supplement regimen, consult your healthcare team. They're your best resource for personalized, evidence-based advice.

Seek reputable sources: When searching for information about kidney health, look for reputable sources like government health agencies, well-established medical organizations, and peer-reviewed research.

Beware of sensational claims: If something sounds too good to be true, it probably is. Be skeptical of products or plans that promise miracle cures or instant results.

Share your findings: If you come across new information or potential scams, share your findings with your healthcare team and fellow kidney patients. Together, we can build a strong, informed community that supports one another in navigating the sea of kidney myths and scams.

Remember, navigating the kidney health maze can be challenging, but with the right tools, a bit of due diligence, and a touch of skepticism, you can steer clear of misinformation and focus on science-based advice that truly benefits your kidney journey.

12 BAD HABITS THAT CAN DAMAGE YOUR KIDNEYS

1. Smoking: Smoking damages blood vessels, impairs blood flow to the kidneys, and accelerates kidney function decline. To avoid kidney damage, quit smoking and seek support from healthcare professionals, smoking cessation programs, and nicotine replacement therapies.

2. Excessive alcohol consumption: Heavy drinking can cause kidney damage and increase the risk of high blood pressure, a leading cause of kidney disease. Limit alcohol consumption to moderate levels (1 drink per day for women, 2 drinks per day for men) or consider abstaining altogether.

3. Overusing painkillers and NSAIDs: Regular use of over-the-counter pain medications, such as ibuprofen and naproxen, can harm the kidneys, especially when taken in high doses or for extended periods. Talk to your healthcare provider about alternative pain management strategies and use these medications only as directed.

4. Consuming too much sodium: A high-sodium diet can raise blood pressure and harm the kidneys. Limit sodium intake by eating fresh, unprocessed

foods, using herbs and spices for flavor, and checking food labels for sodium content.

5. Not managing diabetes: Uncontrolled blood sugar levels can cause kidney damage over time. Monitor blood glucose levels regularly, follow a diabetes-friendly diet, and adhere to your prescribed medication regimen to protect your kidneys.

6. Ignoring high blood pressure: High blood pressure damages blood vessels in the kidneys and can lead to kidney disease. Monitor your blood pressure, follow a heart-healthy diet, exercise regularly, and take prescribed medications to manage high blood pressure.

7. Being sedentary: A lack of physical activity can contribute to obesity, high blood pressure, and type 2 diabetes—all risk factors for kidney disease. Engage in regular physical activity, such as walking, swimming, or yoga, to maintain a healthy weight and support kidney function.

8. Poor hydration: Dehydration can harm the kidneys and increase the risk of kidney stones. Drink adequate amounts of water daily, and adjust your fluid intake based on your healthcare provider's recommendations.

9. Consuming too much protein: A high-protein diet can strain the kidneys, especially in those with kidney disease. Work with a dietitian to determine the appropriate amount of protein for your individual needs and opt for plant-based protein sources when possible.

10. Not getting enough sleep: Chronic sleep deprivation can contribute to high blood pressure and other health problems that affect kidney

function. Establish a consistent sleep schedule, create a relaxing bedtime routine, and prioritize 7-8 hours of sleep each night.

11. Delaying medical care: Ignoring symptoms or delaying medical care for kidney-related issues can lead to further damage. Seek prompt medical attention for concerning symptoms and attend regular check-ups with your healthcare team to address potential issues early.

12. Neglecting mental health: Stress, anxiety, and depression can negatively impact kidney health and overall well-being. Practice stress-reduction techniques, such as meditation, deep breathing exercises, or counseling, and seek professional help when necessary.

By avoiding these harmful habits and adopting a healthy lifestyle, you can protect your kidneys and reduce the risk of kidney disease progression.

UNVEILING MY SECRET TO KIDNEY SUCCESS

Throughout this book, we've explored the complexities of kidney disease, and it's natural to feel overwhelmed at times. But now, let's bring it all together and reveal the secret to my success in managing CKD with a positive and empowering attitude. This is the chapter that will inspire you and prepare you to take charge of your kidney health.

First and foremost, my top priority has been achieving and **maintaining optimal blood pressure** of 120/80 or better and reducing the risk of heart disease. With persistence and teamwork alongside my healthcare providers, we found the right mix of medications for me.

When it comes to the often-confusing task of figuring out what to eat—or more specifically, how much of what to eat—keep in mind that there is no one-size-fits-all diet. It took me well over a year to learn to cook meals and reduce my reliance on pre-made meals. But I learned to view my diet in a different way, and it allowed me to take control and feel confident in my choices.

Think of your diet as a smooth road you want to travel. When your body is missing something, potholes form, making your journey bumpy and slow. By examining my latest lab results, I can identify what's causing these potholes and fix them by adjusting my diet. If necessary, my healthcare team or dietitian might recommend supplements to further support my body.

At times, my body may have too much of something, creating speed bumps that are just as problematic as potholes. In these situations, I adjust my diet or supplements to eliminate the excess and smooth the path ahead. Portion control is essential for a kidney-friendly diet. Your lab results serve as your roadmap, and a dietitian can help you establish daily goals. Then, you're free to choose what you eat throughout the day while staying on track. Free food-tracking apps, like Cronometer (http://go.dadvicetv.com/app), make this even more manageable. This method lets you enjoy a wide variety of foods, including some you never thought possible!

To illustrate this approach, let's use a real-world example. My latest labs reveal that my Potassium is 5.6 (normal range: 3.5 to 5.3) and my Sodium is 132 (normal range: 135 to 146), while everything else appears good. To address these imbalances, I need to slightly reduce my daily potassium target—maybe by eliminating one banana from my daily meal plan. On the other hand, my sodium levels are low, so I can increase my daily sodium target. Since I'm removing the banana, I might also want to increase my fiber intake to make up for the lost fiber. I can add more fiber-rich foods to my diet or consider taking a fiber supplement. It's all about finding balance based on the nutritional targets set by my dietitian. These small, manageable changes should bring my Potassium and Sodium levels within the normal range by my next lab tests.

It's crucial to remember that everyone makes mistakes with their diet, but don't let these setbacks discourage you. If you happen to eat too much of something today, you can adjust for it tomorrow. Your diet isn't restricted to just one day – it's about achieving balance over time. Diet is just one part of the overall strategy for living a fulfilling life with kidney disease. Surround yourself with positivity and avoid people who criticize your food choices. We're all unique, and our food choices will differ – that doesn't mean they're wrong or bad.

Next, managing symptoms and risk factors becomes the third priority. With blood pressure under control and a nutrient-balanced diet, symptoms are minimized or even eliminated. For any lingering issues, I collaborate with my healthcare team to find lifestyle changes or medications to address them. For those with protein in their urine, this is where your healthcare team will work to reduce that, often by incorporating an Ace or Arb medication.

Embracing this positive and confident strategy has transformed my life with kidney disease. I can dine out and enjoy social gatherings without fear, knowing how to make adjustments to keep my diet on track. Portion control allows me to savor almost anything, from a couple of slices of pizza with friends to other favorite dishes. This is the secret that has empowered me to live a full, happy life with kidney disease, and now, it's yours to embrace too.

By adopting this mindset and taking these practical steps, you too can take control of your kidney health and continue to enjoy the foods you love while maintaining a kidney-friendly lifestyle. It's important to note that we all have unique health, lifestyle, and nutritional needs, so our food choices may vary. Trust yourself and your healthcare team to make the best decisions for your individual circumstances.

Living a great life with kidney disease involves a combination of blood pressure management, an individualized, heart-healthy diet, and addressing symptoms or risk factors. Remember to be patient with yourself and stay focused on your goals. With the right mindset and support, you can not only manage but thrive with kidney disease. So, stay positive, stay motivated, and embrace the journey to better kidney health.

EMPOWERING YOURSELF THROUGH KNOWLEDGE AND SUPPORT

Coping with chronic kidney disease (CKD) can be a challenge, but the right information and support resources can significantly enhance the management of the condition and your overall quality of life. This chapter presents a comprehensive list of resources designed to empower individuals with CKD, providing the necessary tools to continue learning about their condition, find support, and stay informed about the latest advancements in CKD care.

Educate and Inspire: Online Resources

DadviceTV.com: This outstanding resource offers invaluable video interviews about kidney disease and its successful management. With expert insights, practical advice, and motivational content, DadviceTV.com helps those with CKD better understand their condition, learn effective management strategies, and stay inspired on their journey to improved kidney health.

PlantPoweredKidneys.com: An amazing and supportive website focused on spreading the word about evidence-based nutrition information for those with chronic kidney disease. Jen Hernandez has a team of renal dietitian nutritionists that provide support, positivity, and motivation. Don't miss Jen's informative Facebook group – it's an excellent resource for meal ideas and positive support.

KidneyNutritionInstitute.org: An organization that aims to provide evidence-based, scientifically rigorous, and unbiased information on nutrition and kidney health. Their primary mission is to advance the understanding of the role of nutrition in the prevention and management of kidney disease. The KNI focuses on research, education, and collaboration to improve the lives of those affected by kidney disease.

UrbanKidneyAlliance.org: A vital resource dedicated to advocate, educate, enlighten, empower, and consult communities and individuals in urban cities at-risk for chronic kidney disease (CKD) and other health-related conditions. Since its inception, Urban Kidney Alliance has helped numerous patients suffering from kidney dialysis with transportation, utility, medication, and nutritional assistance.

American Kidney Fund (AKF): A leading nonprofit organization dedicated to providing support, education, and resources to people affected by kidney disease. With a focus on prevention, early detection, and treatment, the AKF offers financial assistance to patients in need, funds research, and advocates for policies that improve kidney care. Additionally, the organization raises awareness about kidney disease, helping to educate the public on risk factors and promoting healthy lifestyles to prevent the development of kidney-related issues.

National Kidney Foundation (NKF): As a leading authority on kidney health, the NKF provides a wealth of educational materials, webinars, and online courses. Visit their website at kidney.org to access these empowering resources.

American Association of Kidney Patients (AAKP): This patient-centered organization is dedicated to improving the lives of those affected by kidney disease. Offering educational resources, advocacy initiatives, and support services, AAKP is an essential resource for individuals with CKD and their families. Learn more at aakp.org.

Kidney Disease: Improving Global Outcomes (KDIGO): KDIGO's mission is to develop and implement evidence-based clinical practice guidelines for kidney disease. Their website, kdigo.org, offers access to these guidelines, as well as additional resources and educational materials.

Connect and Share: Support Groups and Communities

Local support groups: Connect with others facing similar challenges by joining a local support group. These groups offer a safe space to share experiences, learn from one another, and form lasting connections. Reach out to local hospitals, dialysis centers, or nephrology clinics for information on available support groups in your area.

Online communities: Numerous online forums and communities provide a platform for individuals with CKD to connect with others, ask questions, and share experiences. Popular online platforms include the National Kidney Foundation's community forums (kidney.org/atoz/content/community-forums) and the Davita Kidney Disease and Dialysis Forums (forums.davita.com).

Social media: Social media platforms like Facebook, Twitter, and Instagram offer opportunities to connect with others affected by kidney disease, stay informed about the latest news and research, and access educational content. Follow reputable organizations, healthcare professionals, and patient advocates to engage with and learn from their experiences.

Discover and Grow: Books and Publications

Kidney Disease Cookbooks: Specialized cookbooks cater to the dietary needs of individuals with kidney disease, providing an invaluable resource for kidney-friendly meal planning and delicious recipes. Some popular titles include "Renal Diet

Cookbook for the Newly Diagnosed," "The Kidney Disease Cookbook," and "The Kidney-Friendly Kitchen."

Books on CKD Management: Comprehensive guides on managing CKD and improving kidney health can be found in titles like "**Learn the Facts About Kidney Disease**," "Coping with Kidney Disease," and "Kidney Health Gourmet."

Medical Journals and Publications: Access to peer-reviewed medical journals and publications offers insight into the latest research and advancements in CKD care. Notable journals in the field include the American Journal of Kidney Diseases, the Clinical Journal of the American Society of Nephrology, and Kidney International. Online access to these journals may require a subscription or access through a healthcare professional or institution.

Engage and Learn: Workshops and Conferences

Patient Education Workshops: Many hospitals, clinics, and organizations offer educational workshops specifically designed for individuals with CKD and their families. These workshops cover a variety of topics, including diet and nutrition management, understanding medications, and navigating the healthcare system.

Professional Conferences: Attending professional conferences related to kidney health can provide valuable information on the latest advancements in CKD care, as well as opportunities to network with healthcare professionals and other individuals with kidney disease. Examples of such conferences include the National Kidney Foundation's Spring Clinical Meetings and the American Society of Nephrology's Kidney Week.

Collaborate and Thrive: Healthcare Professionals and Support Services

Nephrologists: Developing a strong relationship with a nephrologist, a physician specializing in kidney care, is crucial for managing CKD. A nephrologist can help create an individualized care plan, monitor kidney function, and adjust treatments as necessary.

Primary Care Physicians (PCP): Regular appointments with a primary care physician can help manage overall health and address potential issues that may impact kidney function.

Registered Dietitians: A registered dietitian with expertise in kidney disease can provide personalized guidance on diet and nutrition, empowering individuals with CKD to make informed choices about their food intake. Working with a dietitian is hands down one of the best decisions you can make to help your kidneys.

Mental Health Professionals: Managing the emotional challenges of living with CKD can be made easier with the support of therapists or counselors, who can help address stress, anxiety, and depression.

Social Workers: Social workers can provide assistance with navigating the healthcare system, accessing financial resources, and connecting with community support services.

Empower and Advocate: Advocacy and Financial Assistance

Patient Advocacy Organizations: Organizations like the National Kidney Foundation and the American Association of Kidney Patients advocate for improved care, increased research funding, and better access to resources for individuals with CKD.

Financial Assistance Programs: Managing CKD can be costly, but many organizations offer financial assistance programs to help cover the expenses related to CKD care. These programs may provide assistance with medication costs, transportation to medical appointments, or other expenses. Examples include the American Kidney Fund and the National Kidney Foundation's Patient Emergency Assistance Program.

By utilizing these resources and surrounding yourself with a supportive network of healthcare professionals, fellow patients, and advocates, you can face the challenges of living with chronic kidney disease with confidence and optimism.

GLOSSARY OF TERMS AND DEFINITIONS

Here's an extensive glossary of kidney-related terms and definitions to help readers familiarize themselves with the language of CKD:

Acidosis: A condition characterized by an excess of acid in the blood, which can cause a variety of symptoms and complications. Acidosis is common in people with kidney disease because the kidneys are responsible for maintaining the body's acid-base balance.

Acute Kidney Injury (AKI): A sudden and temporary loss of kidney function, which can be caused by various factors, such as severe infection, trauma, or medication side effects. AKI can be reversible if treated promptly, but may also lead to chronic kidney disease (CKD) or kidney failure.

Anemia: A condition characterized by a decrease in the number of red blood cells or a decrease in the amount of hemoglobin in the blood. Anemia can cause fatigue, shortness of breath, and other symptoms. It is common in people with kidney disease due to reduced production of the hormone erythropoietin, which stimulates red blood cell production.

Arteriovenous (AV) Fistula: A type of vascular access for hemodialysis that involves connecting an artery directly to a vein, typically in the arm. This creates a high-flow connection that can withstand the pressure of the dialysis machine and provides long-lasting access to the bloodstream.

Automated Peritoneal Dialysis (APD): A form of peritoneal dialysis that uses a machine to automatically exchange the dialysis fluid in the patient's abdominal cavity, typically overnight while the patient sleeps.

Azotemia: A condition characterized by high levels of nitrogen-containing waste products in the blood, such as urea and creatinine. Azotemia can occur in people with reduced kidney function or kidney failure.

Bicarbonate: A substance that helps to neutralize acid in the blood and maintain the body's acid-base balance. People with kidney disease may have low bicarbonate levels, leading to acidosis.

Catheter: A type of vascular access for hemodialysis that involves inserting a long, thin tube (catheter) into a large vein, usually in the neck or chest. Catheters are generally used as a temporary access option when a fistula or graft is not available or is not functioning properly. They have a higher risk of infection and other complications compared to fistulas and grafts.

Chronic Kidney Disease (CKD): A long-term condition characterized by the gradual loss of kidney function over time, which can lead to kidney failure if not treated. CKD can be caused by a variety of factors, such as diabetes, hypertension, and autoimmune diseases.

Continuous Ambulatory Peritoneal Dialysis (CAPD): A form of peritoneal dialysis in which the patient manually exchanges the dialysis fluid in their abdominal cavity several times per day, without the need for a machine.

Creatinine: A waste product that is produced by the normal breakdown of muscle tissue and is removed from the body by the kidneys. Elevated creatinine levels in the blood can be a sign of reduced kidney function.

Dehydration: A condition in which the body does not have

enough water to maintain proper fluid balance and support overall health. Dehydration can cause a variety of symptoms and complications, including kidney damage, and is particularly dangerous for people with kidney disease.

Diabetes: A chronic disease characterized by high blood sugar levels due to the body's inability to produce or effectively use insulin. Diabetes is the leading cause of chronic kidney disease and kidney failure.

Dialysis: A medical treatment that uses a machine to remove waste products and excess fluid from the blood when the kidneys are no longer able to function properly. There are two main types of dialysis: hemodialysis and peritoneal dialysis.

Dialysis Adequacy: A measure of how effectively dialysis is removing waste products and excess fluid from the blood. Adequacy is assessed through regular blood tests and is an important factor in determining the frequency and duration of dialysis treatments.

Diuretics: Medications that help the body get rid of excess fluid by increasing urine production. Diuretics are often used to treat high blood pressure and fluid retention in people with kidney disease.

Donor: A person who provides an organ, such as a kidney, for transplantation. Donors can be living (usually a close relative or friend) or deceased (someone who has died and agreed to donate their organs).

Edema: Swelling caused by excess fluid trapped in the body's tissues, often affecting the legs, ankles, and feet. Edema is a common symptom of kidney disease and can be managed through medications, dietary changes, and other treatments.

Electrolytes: Minerals in the body, such as sodium, potassium, and calcium, that have an electric charge and play crucial roles in maintaining the body's fluid balance, nerve function, and muscle function. Electrolyte imbalances are common in people with kidney disease and can cause a variety of symptoms and complications.

Erythropoiesis-Stimulating Agents (ESAs): Synthetic forms of erythropoietin used to treat anemia in people with kidney disease. These medications stimulate red blood cell production and can help improve symptoms of anemia.

Erythropoietin (EPO): A hormone produced by the kidneys that stimulates the production of red blood cells. People with kidney disease may have reduced EPO production, leading to anemia.

Fistula: A type of vascular access for hemodialysis that involves connecting an artery directly to a vein, typically in the arm. This creates a high-flow connection that can withstand the pressure of the dialysis machine and provides long-lasting access to the bloodstream.

GFR (Glomerular Filtration Rate): A measure of how well the kidneys are filtering waste and excess fluid from the blood. A lower GFR indicates reduced kidney function, with a GFR below 60 considered chronic kidney disease and a GFR below 15 considered kidney failure.

Graft: A type of vascular access for hemodialysis that involves connecting an artery to a vein using a synthetic tube, typically when a fistula is not possible or has failed. Grafts are more prone to infection and clotting than fistulas, but they can provide a reliable access option for some patients.

Hematuria: The presence of blood in the urine, which can be a sign of kidney disease or other medical conditions. Hematuria can be visible to the naked eye (gross hematuria) or only detectable under a microscope (microscopic hematuria).

Hemodialysis: A type of dialysis that uses a machine to filter waste products and excess fluid from the blood through an artificial kidney (dialyzer). Hemodialysis is typically performed in a dialysis center or hospital, usually three times per week.

Hypercalcemia: A condition characterized by high levels of

calcium in the blood. Hypercalcemia can cause a variety of symptoms and complications, including kidney stones and bone disease. It is common in people with advanced kidney disease due to impaired calcium regulation by the kidneys.

Hyperkalemia: A condition characterized by high levels of potassium in the blood. Hyperkalemia can cause muscle weakness, irregular heartbeat, and other symptoms, and can be life-threatening if not treated promptly. It is a common complication of kidney disease and can be managed through diet and medication.

Hyperphosphatemia: A condition characterized by high levels of phosphate in the blood. Hyperphosphatemia is common in people with kidney disease because the kidneys are responsible for filtering excess phosphate from the blood. It can contribute to bone disease and cardiovascular problems.

Hypertension: A condition characterized by consistently high blood pressure, which can damage blood vessels and organs, including the kidneys. Hypertension is both a cause and a complication of kidney disease and requires careful management through lifestyle changes and medications.

Hypocalcemia: A condition characterized by low levels of calcium in the blood. Hypocalcemia can cause muscle cramps, numbness, and other symptoms. It can be a result of certain medications or dietary imbalances and can be managed through diet and supplementation.

Hypokalemia: A condition characterized by low levels of potassium in the blood. Hypokalemia can cause muscle weakness, fatigue, and irregular heartbeat. It can be a result of certain medications or dietary imbalances and can be managed through diet and supplementation.

Hypophosphatemia: A condition characterized by low levels of phosphate in the blood. Hypophosphatemia can cause muscle weakness, bone pain, and other symptoms. It can be a result of certain medications or dietary imbalances and can be managed through diet and supplementation.

IgA Nephropathy: A kidney disease caused by the buildup of the antibody immunoglobulin A (IgA) in the kidneys, leading to inflammation and reduced kidney function. IgA nephropathy is one of the most common causes of glomerulonephritis, and treatment may include medications to manage blood pressure and reduce inflammation.

Kidney Biopsy: A medical procedure in which a small sample of kidney tissue is removed, usually with a needle, for examination under a microscope. A kidney biopsy can help diagnose the cause of kidney disease and guide treatment decisions.

Kidney Failure: The final stage of chronic kidney disease, in which the kidneys are no longer able to filter waste products and excess fluid from the blood. Kidney failure requires treatment with dialysis or a kidney transplant to sustain life.

Kidney Stone: A hard, crystalline mass that forms in the kidneys from substances in the urine, such as calcium, oxalate, and phosphate. Kidney stones can cause severe pain and other symptoms and may require treatment with medications, dietary changes, or surgical intervention.

Kidney Transplant: A surgical procedure in which a healthy kidney from a donor is implanted into a person with kidney failure. A kidney transplant can provide improved quality of life and longer survival compared to dialysis, but it requires lifelong immunosuppressive medications to prevent rejection.

Lupus Nephritis: Kidney inflammation caused by the autoimmune disease lupus, which can lead to kidney damage and reduced kidney function. Treatment for lupus nephritis involves managing the underlying lupus and may include medications to suppress the immune system.

Nephrectomy: The surgical removal of a kidney, usually due to severe damage or cancer. In some cases, a person can live with one functioning kidney, while in others, dialysis or a kidney transplant may be necessary.

Nephritic Syndrome: A group of symptoms and signs caused by inflammation of the glomeruli in the kidneys, leading to reduced kidney function. Nephritic syndrome can include hematuria, hypertension, and reduced urine output.

Nephrologist: A medical specialist who focuses on diagnosing and treating diseases and disorders of the kidneys.

Nephrotic Syndrome: A kidney disorder characterized by high levels of protein in the urine, low levels of protein in the blood, and swelling (edema) due to fluid retention. Nephrotic syndrome can be caused by a variety of underlying conditions, such as diabetes or autoimmune diseases, and can lead to progressive kidney damage if not treated.

Peritoneal Dialysis (PD): A type of dialysis that uses the patient's own peritoneal membrane (lining of the abdominal cavity) as a filter to remove waste products and excess fluid from the blood. PD is typically performed at home, with the patient manually or automatically exchanging dialysis fluid in their abdominal cavity.

Polycystic Kidney Disease (PKD): A genetic disorder that causes numerous fluid-filled cysts to form in the kidneys, leading to enlarged kidneys and reduced kidney function. PKD is the most common inherited cause of kidney disease and can eventually lead to kidney failure.

Potassium: An electrolyte that plays a crucial role in maintaining the body's fluid balance, nerve function, and muscle function. Potassium levels must be carefully managed in people with kidney disease, as both high and low levels can cause serious complications.

Proteinuria: The presence of excess protein in the urine, which can be a sign of kidney disease or other medical conditions. Proteinuria can cause foamy urine and may require treatment with medications or dietary changes.

Renal: Pertaining to the kidneys.

Renal Diet: A specialized diet designed for people with kidney disease, which typically involves controlling the intake of sodium, potassium, phosphorus, and protein to help manage symptoms and slow the progression of kidney disease.

Renal Osteodystrophy: A bone disorder that occurs in people with chronic kidney disease, caused by imbalances in calcium, phosphorus, and parathyroid hormone. Renal osteodystrophy can lead to weak, brittle bones and may require treatment with medications and dietary changes.

Sodium: An electrolyte that plays a crucial role in maintaining the body's fluid balance, nerve function, and muscle function. Sodium levels must be carefully managed in people with kidney disease, as both high and low levels can cause serious complications.

Transplant: A surgical procedure in which a healthy organ from a donor is implanted into a person with organ failure. A kidney transplant is a treatment option for people with kidney failure that can provide improved quality of life and longer survival compared to dialysis.

Urea: A waste product that is produced by the breakdown of proteins in the body and is removed by the kidneys. Elevated levels of urea in the blood can be a sign of reduced kidney function.

Uremia: A condition characterized by high levels of waste products in the blood, such as urea and creatinine, due to reduced kidney function or kidney failure. Uremia can cause a variety of symptoms and complications, including fatigue, nausea, and shortness of breath.

Urinalysis: A laboratory test that examines the chemical and microscopic properties of a urine sample to help diagnose kidney disease and other medical conditions.

Urinary Tract Infection (UTI): An infection in any part of the urinary system, including the kidneys, bladder, or urethra. UTIs are more common in people with kidney disease and can cause pain, fever, and other symptoms.

Urine Output: The amount of urine produced by the kidneys, which can be used to assess kidney function and hydration status. Reduced urine output can be a sign of kidney disease, dehydration, or other medical conditions.

Vascular Access: A method of connecting a patient's bloodstream to a dialysis machine, allowing for the removal of waste products and excess fluid. Common types of vascular access for hemodialysis include arteriovenous fistulas, grafts, and catheters.

Vascular Calcification: and can contribute to cardiovascular complications, such as high blood pressure, heart disease, and stroke. Management of vascular calcification in kidney disease may involve medications, dietary changes, and addressing other risk factors, such as high blood pressure and diabetes.

Vasculitis: Inflammation of the blood vessels, which can cause them to narrow, weaken, or leak. Vasculitis can affect the kidneys and other organs, leading to reduced kidney function or kidney failure. Treatment for vasculitis may include medications to reduce inflammation and suppress the immune system.

Vitamin D: A fat-soluble vitamin that plays a crucial role in maintaining healthy bones, immune function, and overall health. People with kidney disease often have low levels of vitamin D due to impaired kidney function and may require supplementation or treatment with activated vitamin D to maintain normal levels.

Water Intake: The amount of water consumed by a person, which can affect kidney function and overall health. People with kidney disease may need to carefully manage their water intake to prevent dehydration or fluid overload, depending on their individual needs and stage of kidney disease.

Water Retention: The accumulation of excess fluid in the body, often causing swelling (edema) in the legs, ankles, and feet. Water retention is a common symptom of kidney disease and can be managed through medications, dietary changes, and other treatments.

ABOUT THE AUTHOR

James Fabin

James Fabin is a devoted husband and loving father of two young children. Throughout his life, James has been an active participant in charitable endeavors, dedicating his time and resources to make a positive impact on the lives of others.

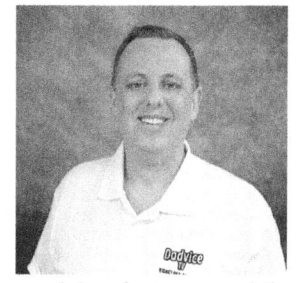

A passionate animal lover, James shares his home with two beloved dogs and volunteers with animal rescue groups, providing support and assistance to animals in need. His dedication to helping others, whether they have two legs or four, is evident in everything he does.

In his professional life, James works in the automotive industry, where he specializes in marketing. His expertise in this field has allowed him to connect with people from all walks of life and apply his skills to create meaningful and lasting relationships.

James's journey with chronic kidney disease has inspired him to share his knowledge and experience with others, providing valuable insights and practical advice through his writing. By combining his passion for helping others with his personal experiences, James hopes to empower those facing kidney disease to take control of their health and improve their quality of life.

Learn more about James and watch his ever-growing kidney video library at www.DadviceTV.com

Made in the USA
Coppell, TX
13 June 2023